Gynecologic Resectoscopy

GENERAL SERIES EDITORS

Eric J. Bieber, M.D.
The University of Chicago
Department of Obstetrics and Gynecology
The Chicago Lying-in Hospital
Chicago, Illinois

Franklin D. Loffer, M.D.
Gynecological Associates, Ltd.
Phoenix, Arizona

FORTHCOMING BOOKS IN THE SERIES:

*Laparoscopic Hysterectomy and
Pelvic Floor Reconstruction,*
edited by C.Y. Liu

The Myomectomy,
edited by E.J. Bieber
and V. Macklin

MINIMALLY INVASIVE GYNECOLOGY SERIES

The Gynecologic Resectoscope

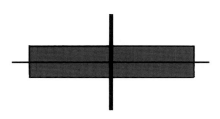

edited by

Eric J. Bieber, M.D.
The University of Chicago
Department of Obstetrics and Gynecology
The Chicago Lying-in Hospital
Chicago, Illinois

Franklin D. Loffer, M.D.
Gynecological Associates, Ltd.
Phoenix, Arizona

b
Blackwell
Science

Blackwell Science

EDITORIAL OFFICES:
238 Main Street, Cambridge, Massachusetts 02142, USA
Osney Mead, Oxford OX2 0EL, England
25 John Street, London WC1N 2BL, England
23 Ainslie Place, Edinburgh EH3 6AJ, Scotland
54 University Street, Carlton, Victoria 3053, Australia
Arnette Blackwell SA, 1 rue de Lille, 75007 Paris, France
Blackwell Wissenschafts-Verlag GmbH, Kurfürstendamm 57, 10707 Berlin,
  Germany
Blackwell MZV, Feldgasse 13, A-1238 Vienna, Austria

DISTRIBUTORS:
North America
    Blackwell Science, Inc.
    238 Main Street
    Cambridge, Massachusetts 02142
    (Telephone orders: 800-215-1000 or 617-876-7000)
Australia
    Blackwell Science Pty Ltd
    54 University Street
    Carlton, Victoria 3053
    (Telephone orders: 03-347-5552)
Outside North America and Australia
    Blackwell Science, Ltd.
    c/o Marston Book Services, Ltd.
    P.O. Box 87
    Oxford OX2 0DT
    England
    (Telephone orders: 44-865-791155)

Acquisitions: Michael Snider
Development: Gail S. Segal
Production: Kathleen Grimes
Typeset by Huron Valley Graphics, Ann Arbor, MI
Printed and bound by BookCrafters, Inc., Chelsea, MI

© **1995 by Blackwell Science, Inc.**

Printed in the United States of America
95 96 97 98 5 4 3 2 1

Library of Congress Cataloging in Publication Data

Gynecologic resectoscopy / edited by Eric J. Bieber, Franklin D.
  Loffer.
      p.   cm. —(Minimally invasive gynecology series)
    Includes bibliographical references and index.

    1. Uterus—Endoscopic surgery.   2. Resectoscopy.   I. Bieber, Eric
J.   II. Loffer, Franklin D.   III. Series.
    [DNLM: 1. Hysteroscopy—methods.   2. Uterine Diseases—diagnosis.
3. Uterine Diseases—surgery.   WP 468 G997 1995]
RG390.G95   1995
618.1′45—dc20
DNLM/DLC
for Library of Congress   94-24319
                                                                      CIP

Contents

Contributors

Randall Barnes, M.D.
The University of Chicago
Department of Obstetrics and
   Gynecology
The Chicago Lying-in Hospital
Chicago, Illinois

Eric J. Bieber, M.D.
The University of Chicago
Department of Obstetrics and
   Gynecology
The Chicago Lying-in Hospital
Chicago, Illinois

Philip G. Brooks, M.D.
UCLA School of Medicine
Cedar-Sinai Medical Center
Los Angeles, California

Richard J. Gimpelson, M.D.
St. Louis University School of
   Medicine
Department of Obstetrics and
   Gynecology
St. Louis, Missouri

Seth Levrant, M.D.
The Center for Human
   Reproduction
Chicago, Illinois

Franklin D. Loffer, M.D.
Gynecological Associates, Ltd.
Phoenix, Arizona

Kevin Loughlin, M.D.
Department of Urology
Brigham and Women's
   Hospital
Boston, Massachusetts

Adam Magos, M.D.
The Royal Free Hospital
London, United Kingdom

Robert S. Neuwirth, M.D.
Columbia University
St. Luke's–Roosevelt Hospital
New York, New York

Richard M. Soderstrom, M.D.
Reproductive Health
    Specialists, P.S.
Seattle, Washington

**Robert D. Tucker, M.D.,
    Ph.D.**
The University of Iowa
College of Medicine
Department of Pathology
Iowa City, Iowa

Rafael F. Valle, M.D.
Northwestern Memorial
    Hospital
Chicago, Illinois

Thierry Vancaillie, M.D.
University of Texas Health
    Sciences Center
San Antonio, Texas

Foreword

The practice of hysteroscopy has added a new dimension to diagnostic and therapeutic gynecology. Twenty years ago the technique became, after a century of incubation, a new method in clinical gynecology. Following the development of improved endoscopes and lighting systems the uterine distension systems were refined and the result was a reliable, reproducible diagnostic method. The initial experiences were of course diagnostic and their clinical relevance at the time was questioned and discussed. Pitfalls and dangers, such as the consequences of intravasation of distension media, were described and indeed remain serious risks of almost all forms of hysteroscopy.

The hysteroscope opened up a new world to gynecology, the interior of the uterus. This included the anatomy, the vasculature and the mucosa; the pathology such as submucous myomata, polyps, endometrial scars; the response to injury seen after division of a septum. Submucous myomectomy or endometrial ablation were removed from the pathology laboratory to the operating room and fell under direct observation of the gynecologist. More specific diagnosis and treatment became possible and gynecologists flocked to postgraduate courses to learn about the new instruments, the new observations about the uterine chamber, and the possibilities of new therapies. As with anything new there were many variations of techniques, varieties of equipment and variable results. For example the initial enthusiasm for hysteroscopic tubal sterilization died down when the results were disappointing, and when the use of the laser for intrauterine surgery, at first very important, had become a secondary method. All of the experiences have expanded our knowledge but have also exposed our ignorance in many areas such as the relationship of submucous myomas to infertility, the natural history of leiomyomata left untreated until the menopause, and the repair processes in the endometrium in response to thermal and mechanical injury. The application of the resectoscope to gynecology was first reported in 1976. Since that time it has gained recognition as a very useful instrument in several conditions and many gynecologists have taken up its use. A central reference source has been lacking.

In this text devoted to the Gynecologic Resectoscope Drs. Eric Bieber and Frank Loffer have assembled a group of contributors respected for their experience and skills with the resectoscope as applied to female reproductive tract disorders. This text offers comprehensive information on the resectoscope, including its history, design, and the principles and function of the interactive components: optics, fluid distension, lighting, electrosurgery, and hazards. The several clinical contributions add considerably to the chapters on basic science with "pearls" on the utilization of the resectoscope in gynecology. In these clinical chapters the concordance and discordance of opinion and experience help to distinguish between what is well established and what is still evolving in our knowledge of intrauterine surgery.

Hysteroscopic surgery is a new area and the resectoscope appears to be the most promising instrument for many of its indications. Therefore gynecologists, like urologists, will require familiarity with it. Since the resectoscope in urology has had a longer history, its place is more clearly defined than the resectoscope in gynecology. Nevertheless, as an interventional instrument for the gynecologist the resectoscope is sure to stay. This text will be an excellent and comprehensive source of information for the practicing gynecologist interested in its use.

Robert S. Neuwirth, M.D.
May 1994

Preface

Hysteroscopy first achieved limited interest amongst gynecologists in the early 1970s when it was thought that it might be able to replace laparoscopy as an effective method of female sterilization. The electrical techniques in use at that time had several disadvantages that resulted in its abandonment.

The second spurt of enthusiasm for learning hysteroscopy occurred in the early 1980s when the formed-in-place silicone plug was being investigated. Although this successful technique is available in Europe, its lack of availability in the United States has resulted in no continuing interest in hysteroscopic sterilization techniques in this country. About this same time, the ability to ablate the endometrial cavity for the control of menorrhagia using Nd:Yag laser energy was published. The enthusiasm that followed this technique further increased interest in hysteroscopy.

However, it was the introduction of the resectoscope and electrical energy to perform intrauterine surgery that has resulted in the most recent and wide-spread increased interest in diagnostic and operative hysteroscopy. The ready availability of electricity as an energy source in virtually all hospitals and the ability to pattern some form of treatment after the experience of urologists, has made this technique available to most experienced hysteroscopists.

The division of the subject into the chapters we have selected is certainly arbitrary. There inevitably is a cross over between chapters of techniques, theoretical considerations, and procedures. However, we selected contributing authors who could act as spokesmen for the technique described. They were asked to provide not only a manual as to accomplishing the procedure but the rationale and results based on the procedure. In this fashion it is hoped that the reader will be able to achieve a balanced view of the value and uses of the resectoscope. Inevitably in a multi-authored text there might initially appear to be conflicting opinions. Rather than confusing the reader; this should simply alert them that there are generally several ways of accomplishing the same goal.

Undoubtedly some of the more difficult and complex intrauterine surgical procedures will eventually be done by a limited number of hysteroscopists. However, it is our belief that all gynecologists should be capable of evaluating the uterine cavity by hysteroscopy and accomplishing the more common and simpler intrauterine surgical procedures.

We hope that this text will allow those experienced in diagnostic hysteroscopy to advance their skills in hysteroscopic/resectoscopic intrauterine surgery.

Eric J. Bieber, M.D.
Franklin D. Loffer, M.D.

Acknowledgments

It was our hope when this book was conceived that it would provide a source for practicing gynecologic endoscopists who are using or wish to use the resectoscope. It is clear as one reviews the literature on intrauterine surgery that electrical energy has assumed increasing importance and is more versatile than either mechanical or laser energy.

We intended that this text provide not only a manual of instruction in order to perform resectoscopic surgery, but also to present the theoretical considerations that lead to variation in techniques. It would have been impossible to accomplish this without the expertise, wisdom and skill of our contributors. We are indeed appreciative for their sharing these with our readers.

Others also have made this text possible. Gail S. Segal, the developmental editor at Blackwell, and Lee Medoff, the production editor, have allowed us a smooth interface with the publication of this material. In addition we each must acknowledge our personal staff's contributions, Marilyn Harter's help in researching material has been invaluable, as has Carole Jones' and Judy Runges' untiring efforts in preparation of the manuscripts.

Finally, we wish to express our appreciation and love to our wives, Edie Bieber and Trish Loffer, and families, who tolerated the months of clutter in our studies and the hours of absence amongst that clutter.

MINIMALLY INVASIVE GYNECOLOGY SERIES

Gynecologic Resectoscopy

1

The Origins of the Resectoscope

Kevin R. Loughlin

T here are several reasons why a knowledge and understanding of the origins of the resectoscope should be important to the modern surgeon. First, the resectoscope is one of the most common surgical instruments in use today. In 1989, over 400,000 transurethral resections of the prostate were performed (1). Its use in gynecology has significantly increased over the last decade. Second, the same skepticism and uncertainty that surrounds many aspects of surgical innovation today were present during the development of the resectoscope. It should give us perspective to recall what was said in a textbook of urology over 35 years ago,

> Despite the extensive salesmanship with which transurethral resection was promoted in the early 1930s as a simple, successful operation without important danger, the procedure has suffered greatly at the hands of both trained and untrained blunderers with an overall mortality and morbidity in excess of open operation. Yet, today, in the hands of the competent, the mortality is not over two to four percent in all cases, hemorrhage and infection being the grave and relating frequent complications. Bleeding may occur weeks or even months

postoperatively. Transurethral resection is decidedly an operation only for expert experienced hands (2).

The resectoscope, like most significant surgical advances, cannot be credited to one individual. The development of the resectoscope was the culmination of the independent as well as joint efforts of basic scientists and clinicians to solve a surgical problem. The genesis of the resectoscope can best be credited to the work of Bottini, who in 1877 described his galvanocautery incisor. His incisor was fitted with a platinum blade and connected to a source of electricity using insulated wires. However, Bottini's instrument did not permit the surgeon any visualization of the obstructive lesion. Modifications of Bottini's instrument were made by Freudenberg, Goldschmidt, Wishard, and Chetwood, but none of their designs achieved widespread acceptance (3).

Nesbit credits the development of the resectoscope to three discoveries: the incandescent lamp, high frequency current, and the fenestrated sheath (3). Thomas Edison invented the incandescent lamp in 1879 and within a decade duRocher had constructed a cystoscope that incorporated the incandescent lamp.

In 1900, the first American-made cystoscope was designed by Reinhold Wappler and William Otis in New York and was presented at the American Association for Genito-Urinary Surgeons in 1900 (3). Early contributions and continued modifications of the resectoscope were made by Hugh Young, William Braasch, and Bransford Lewis. However, the next major advance in resectoscope design belongs to Maximilian Stern and Joseph McCarthy.

In 1926, Maximilian Stern published an article describing his instrument for transurethral resection of the prostate (4). Stern designed a cutting hoop that consisted of a small ring of tungsten about 0.5 cm in diameter placed at right angles to the end of an insulated shaft. The tungsten loop was positioned in front of the eye of the telescope and was moved backward toward the operator to cut tissue. Stern's original illustrations are reproduced in Figures 1-1 and 1-2. Stern is credited with first using the term "resectoscope".

During the time when the early resectoscopes were undergoing

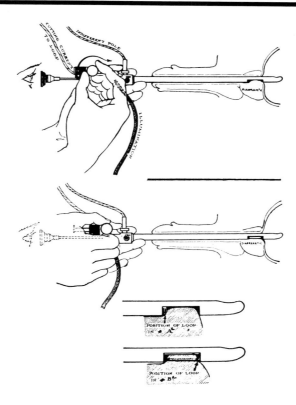

FIGURE 1-1

Stern's resectoscope as it appeared in the *Journal of the American Medical Association,* 1926. (Reproduced by permission from Stern M. Resection of obstructions at the vesical orifice. JAMA 1926;87:1726–1730.)

development, other technological advances were occurring in parallel. A young physicist in Boston, William T. Bovie, was working on the development of a new electrosurgical unit to cauterize tissue. The first time Bovie's unit was used clinically was October 1, 1926, at the Peter Bent Brigham Hospital (5). Harvey Cushing was the operating surgeon and he used Bovie's electrocautery unit to remove a vascular myeloma. Bovie's work made the application of diathermy possible to open surgical procedures. Also, Bovie's investigations into the applications of surgical electrocautery laid the foundation for further refinement of the resectoscope. However, early on, clinical surgeons were skeptical of the electrocautery unit and did not embrace its use.

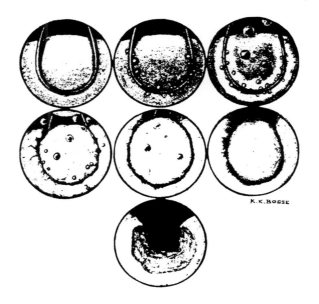

FIGURE 1-2

Stern's resectoscope loop, 1926. (Reproduced by permission from Stern M. Resection of obstructions at the vesical orifice. JAMA 1926;87:1726–1730.)

Bovie ultimately sold his patent for the electrocautery unit to the Liebel–Florsheim Company for one dollar (5).

The early applications of electrical current for transurethral prostate resection were cumbersome. Edward L. Keyes, Jr. and Clyde W. Collings are credited with the first use of cutting electrical current for prostatic obstruction (3). They employed a vacuum tube to supply the current and were unable to use the current underwater, so they distended the bladder with oil (3). They reported their initial experience at the American Urological Association meeting in June, 1924. It was not until 1931, however, that the vacuum tube generator had sufficient power to enable the urologist to cut tissue underwater. A machine using a vacuum tube generator was developed by Frederick Wappler and was marketed by the ACMI company under the name of the Comprex Oscillator (3).

In addition to improvements in optics and electrocautery, the introduction of the fenestrated tube facilitated the development of the resectoscope. Hugh Young first used a fenestrated tube for his

cold punch instrument in 1909 (3). However, Young's original instrument did not permit visualization of the prostate by the surgeon. A few years later, Braasch developed a fenestrated sheath that
incorporated direct visualization. In 1926, Bumpus at the Mayo
Clinic further modified Braasch's instrument by using a tubular
knife connected to high frequency coagulatory current. Bumpus is
credited with designing the first instrument for transurethral resection that incorporated the incandescent lamp, high frequency electrical current, and the fenestrated tube (3).

A North Carolina urologist, Theodore Davis, utilized the
Bovie generation for transurethral resections. Perhaps his major con-
tribution was the development of a magnetic foot switch that en-
abled the operating surgeon himself, rather than an assistant, to turn
the electrical current off and on.

Joseph McCarthy first reported on his new modification of this
resectoscope in a two-page report in the *Journal of Urology* in 1931 (6).
In 1932, McCarthy further modified his resectoscope, which was in

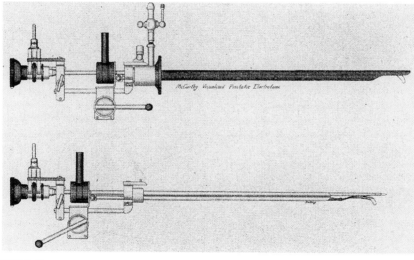

FIGURE 1-3

McCarthy's resectoscope as it appeared in the *New England Journal of Medicine,* 1932. (Reproduced by permission from McCarthy JF. The management of prostatic obstructions by endoscopic revision. N Engl J Med
1932;207(7):305–312.)

reality the forerunner of the modern instrument. His design included a foroblique lens system with magnification as well as a Bakelite sheath for insulation. That year, McCarthy authored a classic article in the *New England Journal of Medicine* entitled "The Management of Prostatic Obstruction by Endoscopic Revision" (7). A picture of McCarthy's instrument appears in Figure 1-3. Further refinement of the resectoscope continued, and Reed Nesbit persuaded Mr. Frederick Wappler, the president of American Cystoscope Makers, Inc., to design a resectoscope that could be used with one hand (3). This would permit the surgeon's other hand to be placed into the O'Conor drape and palpate the prostate transrectally during the resection.

Once the resectoscope became established as a viable surgical instrument, the choice of irrigation fluid became a subject of debate. The early experience with sterile water had resulted in red cell hemolysis and renal failure. Creevy (8) published some of the early

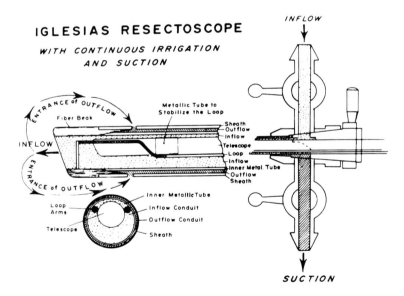

FIGURE 1-4

Iglesias' resectoscope as described in the *Journal of Urology,* 1975. (Reproduced by permission from Iglesias JJ, Sporer A, Gellman AC, Seebode JJ. New Iglesias resectoscope with continuous irrigation, simultaneous suction, and low intravesicle pressure. J Urol 1975;114:929–933.)

1870			
	-	1877	Bottini—galvanocautery incisor
1880	-	1879	Edison—incandescent lamp
1890			
1900	-	1900	Wappler—first American cystoscope
1910	-	1909	Young—fenestrated tube
1920	-	1926	Bovie—electrosurgical unit
		1926	Stern—resectoscope loop
1930	-	1932	McCarthy—foroblique lens
1940			
	-	1947	Creevy—research on irrigating solutions
1950			
1960			
1970			
	-	1975	Iglesias—Continuous irrigation resectoscope
1980			

FIGURE 1-5

Development of the Resectoscope

work using an isotonic (4%) glucose solution as an irrigation fluid in order to prevent hemolysis. Subsequently, most endoscopic resectionists have used either mannitol, sorbitol, or glycine as irrigating solutions. All these solutions are less hypotonic with plasma, and, therefore, do not carry the risk of intravascular hemolysis; however, they can cause hyponatremia.

In 1975, Iglesias and coworkers (9) published a report on their resectoscope, which has emerged as the "modern" resectoscope and is presently used by most surgeons who perform transurethral resections of the prostate. The new Iglesias resectoscope permits simultaneous suction and continuous irrigation, which results in better visualization of the fluid and lower bladder pressure. The design for the Iglesias resectoscope appears in Figure 1-4.

The development of the resectoscope essentially took a century to complete. Multiple individuals, some known and some unknown, contributed to its development. The major events that led to the ultimate creation of the resectoscope appear on the "time line" in Figure 1-5. It would be naive to assume that the refinement of the resectoscope is complete. Undoubtedly, as long as surgeons use a resectoscope to treat patients, they will continue to redesign, modify, and perfect the instrument.

REFERENCES

1. Holtgrewe HL, Mebust WK, Dowd JB, Cockett AT, Peters PC, Proctor C. Transurethral prostatectomy: practice aspects of the dominant operation in American urology. J Urol 1989;141(2):248–253.
2. Campbell MF. Tumors of the urogenital tract. In: Campbell MF, ed. Principles of Urology. Philadelphia: WB Saunders, 1957:444–510.
3. Nesbit RM. A history of transurethral prostatic resection. In: Silber SJ, ed. Transurethral Resection. New York: Appleton-Century-Crofts, 1977:1–17.
4. Stern M. Resection of obstructions at the vesical orifice. JAMA 1926; 87:1726–1730.
5. Goldwyn RM. Bovie: the man and the machine. Ann Plas. Surg 1979; 2(2):135–153.
6. McCarthy JF. A new apparatus for endoscopic plastic surgery of the prostate, diathermia, and excision of vesical growths. J Urol 1931; 26:695–696.
7. McCarthy JF. The management of prostatic obstructions by endoscopic revision. N Engl J Med 1932;207(7):305–312.
8. Creevy CD, Webb EA. A fatal hemolytic reaction following transurethral resection of the prostate gland: a discussion of its prevention and treatment. Surgery 1947;21:56–66.
9. Iglesias JJ, Sporer A, Gellman AC, Seebode JJ. New Iglesias resectoscope with continuous irrigation, simultaneous suction, and low intravesicle pressure. J Urol 1975;114:929–933.

2

Resectoscopic Instrumentation

Seth Levrant

G ynecological resectoscopic surgery is an extension of operative hysteroscopy. The basic principles of operative hysteroscopy apply to resectoscopy. Knowledge of and experience with the basic techniques and instrumentation of diagnostic and operative hysteroscopy are prerequisite to safe and successful resectoscopy. Instruments that are common to hysteroscopy and resectoscopy include: (a) the endoscope (hysteroscope), (b) light source, (c) distention media and irrigation systems, (d) electrosurgical devices, and (e) video camera systems. Unique to resectoscopy is the resectoscope and its electrodes.

RESECTOSCOPE

The gynecologic resectoscope is a modified urological resectoscope having a shorter, blunter insulating beak at its distal end (Figure 2-1). The first reports of gynecological applications of this technique utilized the urological resectoscope (1–4). The gynecologic resectoscope consists of a rigid 3- or 4-mm hysteroscope (telescope), the resectoscope working element, an inner sheath, and an outer sheath (Figure 2-2). The electrodes and the electrosurgical device attach to

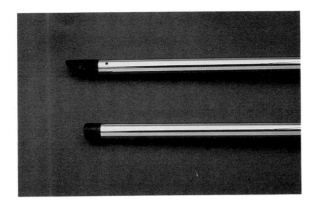

FIGURE 2-1

Gynecological resectoscope (bottom) has shorter, blunter insulating beak than urological resectoscope (top). (Photograph courtesy of Richard Wolf Medical Instruments Corp.)

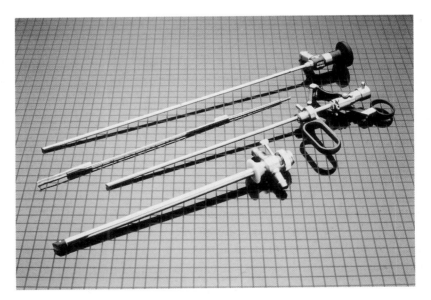

FIGURE 2-2

Telescope, electrode, resectoscope working element, and assembled inner and outer sheaths. (Photograph courtesy of Karl Storz Endoscopy.)

the resectoscope working element, which contains a built-in finger-controlled spring system that moves the electrode forward and back. Gynecologic resectoscopes utilize a passive spring mechanism. The electrode is inside the sheath in the resting position, advances past the sheath against the spring, and then returns to the sheath (during cutting) by the force of the spring. The electrodes move about 3–4 cm within the visual field of the telescope. Electrical current should only be applied to the electrode when the operative site is completely visualized and the electrode is returning to the sheath.

The original resectoscope was a single flow device with only an inflow sheath. This is still available for use with high viscosity distention media. The continuous flow resectoscope provides continuous flushing of low viscosity distention media, resulting in better visualization and safer surgery. The distention media inflow is through the inner sheath and the outflow is through the outer sheath (Figures 2-3, 2-4). The double-channeled sheaths are designed for minimal inflow resistance and have a slightly higher outflow resistance. This resulting continuous flow increases visibility while maintaining intrauterine pressure and distention. The pattern of holes at the distal end of the outer sheath varies by manufacturer (Table 2-1, Figures 2-4, 2-5).

Resectoscopes come in a variety of sizes (Table 2-1). The 24 (8-mm), 25, 26, 27 (9-mm), and 28 French resectoscopes utilize the 4-mm telescope. They have separate inflow and outflow sheaths and open (u shaped) wire loop electrodes. These resectoscopes are used for all aspects of resectoscopic surgery, but are particularly well suited for the resection of submucosal myomas and large polyps. The 21 French (7-mm) resectoscopes utilize the 3-mm telescope. They have one sheath that contains both the inflow and outflow channels, and closed wire loop electrodes. These smaller resectoscopes are well suited for removal of small polyps, lysis of intrauterine adhesions, and lysis of uterine septa. Resectoscopes are 30–35 cm in total length and have working distances of 18–19.5 cm. An extended working length resectoscope (22, 26.5-cm) is available for use in the slightly enlarged uterus (Table 2-1).

TABLE 2-1

Continuous Flow Resectoscopes

Manufacturer	Size	Telescope Size	Viewing Angle	Outer Sheath Outflow Holes	Connector	Features
Circon ACMI	25 Fr	4 mm	12°,30°	top and bottom	snap-in	Bridge to convert resectoscope to operative hysteroscope
	27 Fr	4 mm	12°,30°	top and bottom		Inflow/outflow port on outer sheath
Cooper	27 Fr	4 mm	0°,15°,30°	encircle	rotary/twist	
Karl Storz	21 Fr	2.9 mm	0°	encircle (single row)	rotary/twist	
	*24 Fr	4 mm	0°,12°,30°			Laser fiber channel
	*24 Fr	4 mm	0°,12°,30°			Extended working length (22 and 26.5 cm)
	26 Fr	4 mm	0°,12°,30°	top and bottom		
	28 Fr	4 mm	0°,12°,30°	top and bottom		
Olympus	7 mm	3 mm	0°	top and side	snap-in	
	8 mm	4 mm	0°,12°,30°	top and side		
	9 mm	4 mm	0°,12°,30°	top and side		Optical obturator rotatable sheath
Richard Wolf	24 Fr	4 mm	5°,25°	top	rotary/twist	
	27 Fr	4 mm	5°,25°	top		

*Single channel resectoscopes.

7 mm = 21 Fr (French), 8 mm = 24 Fr, and 9 mm = 27 Fr.

Currently available continuous flow resectoscopes are listed by manufacturer and size (maximum outer sheath diameter). The four basic electrode designs (see Figure 2-7), plus several variations on these designs, are available with 25 Fr and larger resectoscopes. Electrode selection/variety tends to be limited with the smaller resectoscopes; however, this varies with manufacturer and is expected to improve.

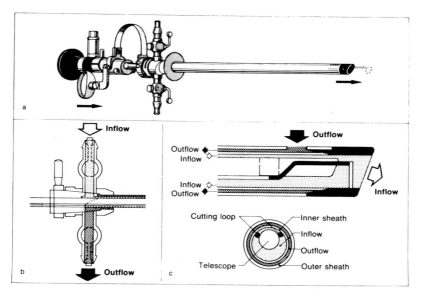

FIGURE 2-3

(a) Resectoscope with continuous flow irrigation. (b) Schematic of in- and outflow channels. (c) Longitudinal section of the instrument tip. Cross-section shows the fluid outflow, which lies between the inner and outer sheaths, the inner tube with telescope, cutting loop connectors, and lumen for inflow irrigating solution. (Reproduced by permission from Matouschek E. Urologic Endoscopic Surgery. St. Louis: Mosby-Year Book, 1989.)

The light cable and distention media inflow attach on the top, and the distention media outflow attaches on the bottom. Reversal of the distention media inflow and outflow attachments will hinder effective intrauterine distention and visibility (Figure 2-3). The electric cable attachment site varies with manufacturer. There are two basic designs for how the instruments lock in place. One is a rotary or twisting lock mechanism, and the other is a snap-in connection (Figures 2-2, 2-6). The rotary design can untwist while rotating the resectoscope during surgery, if one is not careful. The snap-in system will not unlock while rotating the instrument; however, if not held correctly, the resectoscope may unlock when moved within the uterine cavity or removed from the uterine cavity.

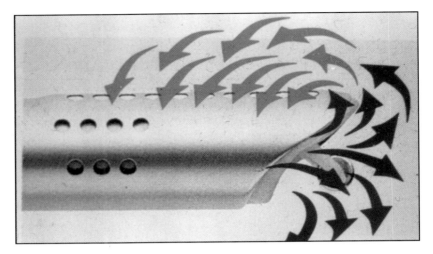

FIGURE 2-4

Distal tip of Olympus 9-mm outer sheath. Note top and sidehole pattern with schematic of intrauterine irrigation flow. (Photograph courtesy of Olympus Corp.)

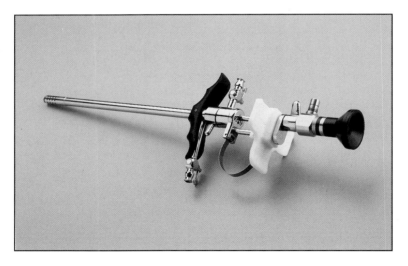

FIGURE 2-5

Cooper Surgical 27 Fr resectoscope. Distal tip of outer sheath has hole pattern that encircles the sheath. (Photograph courtesy of Cooper Surgical, Inc.)

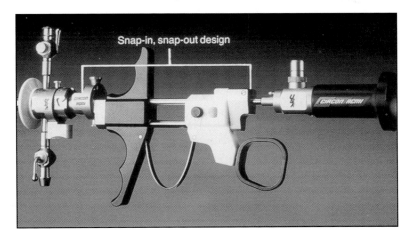

FIGURE 2-6

Resectoscope with snap-in locking mechanism. (Photograph courtesy of Circon ACMI.)

ELECTRODES

There are four basic designs of resectoscopic electrodes: the (a) loop, (b) bar/barrel, (c) ball, and (d) point or knife-like tip (Figure 2-7). The loop electrodes are used primarily to shave or remove myomas and polyps. The 90°, 45°, and 120° loops are well suited for this purpose. The 0° loop and point or knife-like tips can be used for resection of septa or lysis of intrauterine adhesions. Endometrial ablation is performed using either the 90° loop, the ball, the bar/barrel electrode, or some combination of the three. The ball and bar/barrel electrodes increase the electrode surface area, thereby decreasing current density and heating. The depth of coagulation achieved is dependent on the electrode surface area, time of exposure, and the electrical source and power (see Chapter 3) (5).

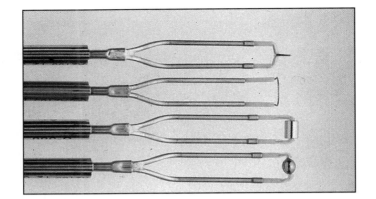

FIGURE 2-7

Basic electrode designs for resectoscopy: point, loop, bar/barrel, and ball. (Photograph courtesy of Olympus Corp.)

TELESCOPES

The same telescopes used for operative hysteroscopy are used with the resectoscope. These are panoramic telescopes with a rod lens optical system and a 3- or 4-mm outer diameter. The telescope is focused at infinity; therefore, the image is smaller than actual size when it is positioned away from the object (6). Magnification is inversely proportional to the distance of the object from the lens (6). The working distance is 30–35 mm, and because hysteroscopes are monocular, there is little depth perception. The panoramic field varies from approximately 70° to 120°, depending on model and manufacturer. Telescopes are available with a viewing angle of 0°, 5°, 12°, 15°, 25°, or 30° (Figure 2-8). The acute angle telescopes (25° and 30° foroblique) are better suited for visualizing the uterine cornua and lateral walls. However, the fully extended electrode may go beyond the field of view when using a 30° telescope. The visual field may be partially blocked by the electrode when using a 0° viewing angle. For general resectoscopic surgery, there is no single angle of vision that is best. Prior to purchasing a resectoscope, you should operate with the different angles of vision to determine

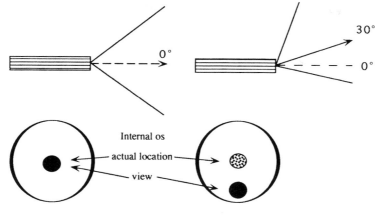

FIGURE 2-8

Field of view between 0° (on left) and 30° foroblique telescope. As the 30° telescope passes through the cervical canal with the telescope's axis of symmetry aimed ventrally (at the symphysis pubis), the internal as appears lower in the field of view than where it actually lies.

which is best. Ideally, operating with each of the different telescopes within the same uterine cavities should be tried.

DISTENTION DEVICES

Intrauterine distention during resectoscopy can be achieved using gravity or a pump. Hanging low viscosity distention media approximately eight feet above the floor (a few feet above the patient) and using wide-bore urological tubing [transurethral prostatic resection (TUR) tubing] has been successfully employed by many surgeons. Standard intravenous (IV) tubing, because of its narrow diameter and high resistance to flow, does not allow a satisfactory distention media flow rate. Standard IV tubing should not be used for resectoscopic surgery. One of the first systems adapted for resectoscopic surgery was a diaphragm pump that used pressurized nitrogen to generate intrauterine pressure and distention media flow.

This pump was removed from the market by the manufacturer due to concerns of the possibility of gas embolism. In the United States, there is currently one irrigation system on the market. This system, the Zimmer CDIS pump®, has an inflow channel pressure sensor. The infusion pressure setting is adjustable to a maximum of 80 mmHg. In Europe, the Hamou Hysteromat and Staflo pumps also have built-in sensors to monitor inflow channel pressure. Still lacking is a way to directly monitor intrauterine pressure. An alternative to using gravity or a pump has been the use of pressure cuffs; however, pressures cannot be regulated very well and there is a tendency for the pressure to drop as the bag empties (7).

In general, flow rates are between 50 and 200 mL/min. Intrauterine pressure should not exceed 80 mmHg. The minimal pressure needed to provide adequate distention and visualization should be used at all times.

ELECTROSURGICAL DEVICES

A high-frequency electrosurgical unit with a digital wattage indicator is preferable to one with arbitrary dial settings. For safer electrosurgery, the electrosurgical unit should be isolated electrically and advantage taken of developments in the return electrode, i.e., the Valleylab Return Electrode Monitoring Circuit (REM), or equivalent. This is discussed in more detail in Chapter 3, with the use of monopolar current.

VIDEO EQUIPMENT

Attaching the video camera to the telescope and performing the surgery while viewing the images on a video monitor magnifies the surgical field, dramatically improves the surgeon's comfort, and allows for greater participation and interest of the operating room staff. The equipment requirements for resectoscopy are the same as those for hysteroscopy and essentially the same as those for laparoscopy.

The basic components include a video camera, high-resolution medical video monitor, video recorder, and color video printer.

Camera

Video camera technology is advancing rapidly with increased resolution, increased light sensitivity, and most importantly, enhanced processing of the video image. Cameras currently used for endoscopy consist of a lens and either one or three solid-state integrated circuit image sensors referred to as CCDs (charge coupled device) or chips. In single-chip cameras, the picture element contains thousands of photosensitive cells, or pixels, that detect either the colors red, green, or blue. In a camera in which one-third of the pixels are devoted to each color, only one-third of the image falls on any given color. The camera circuitry, then, has to generate colors electronically for the areas that fall on the other pixel colors. Three-chip cameras have three picture elements, each devoted to a single color (red, blue, and green), and each sees the entire image. Single-chip cameras have a 20% reduction in pixel resolution as a result of color filtration, but require approximately 15% less light than three-chip cameras. This is changing with increased technology; new three-chip cameras require less light than older single-chip cameras.

Video noise and background graininess, or snow, are measured by the signal-to-noise (S/N) ratio on a logarithmic scale. The higher the S/N ratio, the better the picture. The better single-chip cameras have S/N ratios of around 47 decibels compared to S/N ratios of 60+ decibels for three-chip cameras.

Differences in single-chip camera systems include the camera head and telescopic optics; the color reproduction, tone, and tints are essentially the same. Single-chip cameras come in two sizes, the half-inch chip and the two-thirds-inch chip. The latter has increased resolution (450–550 lines) compared to the former (300–450 lines); 600–800 lines of resolution are generated by three-chip cameras. Three-chip cameras have increased color separation and resolution, and decreased noise, and are almost twice the cost of single-chip camera systems.

Features to look for with any camera include a small, lightweight camera head with focusing ring and zoom feature (usually

25–40 mm) and a camera system that has automatic adjustments for its various features and no more than three buttons. Some of these features include gain control (compensates for reflections of bright images), brightness (shutter) control (regulates light through the light source), color adjustment, and white balance.

Additional advances in camera technology include the "Hyper HAD" charge coupled device (CCD) which improves light sensitivity by capturing the light that falls between pixels and by digital technology. Camera image transmission and processing have traditionally utilized analog technology. Digital processing involves converting the analog wave form to the binary language utilized by computers. Digital signal processing has improved the image quality of the analog camera systems on the market. This is why today's cameras are better than those of just a few years ago. The other advantage of digital processing is that it allows direct communication with other digital technology, i.e., computers and telecommunications, as well as digital image storage. Your surgical images can be stored digitally on a computer disk, or CD, enhanced using computer software, and then printed. The stored image can also be made into slides or transmitted via modem. Advances to look for include the digital camera, which could have the camera chip at the tip of the endoscope, bypassing the traditional optics system entirely, and integrated digital systems that include the VCR, printer, camera, monitor, and computer.

Monitor

The medical monitors found in most operating rooms have about 450–600 lines of resolution. This is all that is needed for the single-chip camera. To take full advantage of the increasing resolution of newer cameras, it is necessary to have a high-resolution medical monitor that has 700+ lines of resolution. Anticipated advances in monitors for include high definition TV and three-dimensional TV imaging.

Light Source

There are a number of options when it comes to light sources. The 150 W lamp with or without flash generator is certainly sufficient for hysteroscopy and resectoscopy. However, the xenon or metal halide light sources are better suited for videotaping and still photography. Xenon light sources can give a bluish color distortion, while metal halides can give a reddish color distortion. However, these color distortions are corrected by most camera systems.

Video Recorder

Video recorders also come in a variety of formats and sizes. The standard VHS recorder has approximately 250 lines of resolution, and the super VHS (S–VHS) recorder has approximately 400 lines of resolution. Both utilize half-inch tape as does the Betacam or Betacam SP system. While the 0.75-inch U-matic SP high-band recording, referred to as BVU, is considered professional quality, the 0.75-inch U-matic low band is considered semiprofessional. When editing is required, either 0.75-inch U-matic format is superior to the 0.5-inch VHS tape systems. However, for routine documentation of endoscopic surgery, a professional grade VHS recorder is sufficient. The 8-mm format (V8) is also available for documentation of hysteroscopic surgery.

Video Standards

There are three major video standards used in the world. The NTSC (National Television Standard Committee) standard is used in North America, Japan, and parts of South America and Asia. The PAL (phase-alternating line) standard is used in Western Europe, Australia, New Zealand, and parts of Africa and the Far East. The SECAM (Séquentiel Couleur a Mémoire) standard is used in France, Eastern Europe, and parts of Africa and Asia. The standards differ in how color is encoded and the number of image lines. PAL and SECAM have 625 image lines compared to 525 lines with NTSC. PAL is more expensive than NTSC but has increased color stability and reproduction. Improved image quality with the NTSC system is achieved with the "Y/C" (luminance–chrominance) output. In the NTSC system, the RGB (red, green, blue) signal is encoded into a single composite. Camera systems with the Y/C output encode the RGB signal electronically into separate luminance (black and white) and chrominance (color) signals but do not encode these two signals into the final composite NTSC signal (8). The resulting image has decreased bleeding of colors and superior quality. The entire video system, from video camera to recorder and then to monitor, must maintain the signal in the Y/C form throughout.

ANCILLARY INSTRUMENTS

Some of the accessory instruments required for diagnostic and operative hysteroscopy are needed for resectoscopy. These include a weighted speculum and vaginal wall retractors or a single-hinged (open-side) speculum, conventional double-tooth tenaculum, and cervical dilators. To remove myoma chips, a myoma-grasping forceps is very useful; however, polyp forceps, pituitary rongeur, ring forceps, or curette can be used instead. When using low viscosity liquid distention media, larger diameter urology tubing should be used. Standard intravenous tubing has a smaller diameter and a much higher resistance to flow. Use of special surgical drapes, which funnel fluids into a drain pouch, are exceedingly important in monitoring input and output during resectoscopy. Many surgeons attach the outflow port of the resectoscope to low pressure suction instead of simply allowing the outflow to drain into the pouch. Because there can be drainage from around the cervix, even when attaching the outflow port directly to suction, surgical drapes that funnel fluid into a pouch should be used. Urologic and neurosurgical drapes were used prior to the design and marketing of gynecological resectoscopic surgical drapes.

OPERATING ROOM SETUP

The operating room should be arranged to minimize clutter and maximize efficiency for the surgeon and nursing staff. Resectoscopy requires the same operating room setup as operative hysteroscopy with the addition of the electrosurgical device and, possibly, an irrigation pump. Arrangement of equipment should be part of the planning before procedures begin. Placement of the video camera cable, light source cable, electrosurgical cable, and distention media input and output tubing need to be considered. In addition, there is the Foley catheter and foot pedal to the electrosurgical unit. If the bottom drape pouch has a valve at the bottom, this and the output tubing may both be connected to suction. If a distention media irrigation system is used, this is an additional piece of equipment whose displays should be clearly visible. A clear and unobstructed view of the video monitor that does not cause the surgeon's neck to strain is essential. This is accomplished with either a monitor near the head of the table or a video cart with a swivel arm for the monitor, or by placing the monitor near the patient's hip with the monitor high on the cart and the patient's hip slightly flexed. Urological or Allen stirrups are better than the traditional candy cane stirrups for these purposes. Generally, the light source, video monitor, and video camera are on one cart; therefore, these three cables will go together in one direction. Placing the irrigation tubing (and device) and electrosurgical unit on the opposite side of the patient usually works best. The surgical assistant or scrub nurse may stand to the side of the surgeon, or on the patient's side, depending on operating room size and personal preference. Either the circulating nurse or anesthesiologist should be assigned to monitor input/output prior to starting the surgery.

The surgeon should have a working knowledge of the video equipment. This should include start-up, basic troubleshooting, and the ability to explain how to record the surgery on the VHS or print pictures using the video printer to someone who has never laid eyes on the equipment. A complete understanding of how to put together the resectoscope and connect the electrodes and cables is essential for hassle-free surgery.

If you do not understand your equipment, you will one day have to explain to your patient that you had to cancel or could not complete her surgery because of technical difficulties (your usual operating room staff called in sick!).

CLINICAL PEARLS

✖ Knowledge of and experience with the basic techniques and instrumentation of diagnostic and operative hysteroscopy are a prerequisite to safe and successful resectoscopy.

✖ The gynecologic resectoscope consists of a rigid 3- or 4-mm hysteroscope (telescope), the resectoscope working element, an inner sheath, and an outer sheath.

✖ Gynecologic resectoscopes utilize a passive spring mechanism. The electrode is inside the sheath in the resting position, advances past the sheath against the spring, and then returns to the sheath (during cutting) by the force of the spring.

✖ Current should only be applied to the electrode when the operative site is completely visualized, the electrode location is known, and the electrode is returning to the sheath.

✖ The continuous flow resectoscope provides continuous flushing of low viscosity distention media, resulting in better visualization and safer surgery.

✖ The smaller resectoscopes are well suited for removal of small polyps, lysis of intrauterine adhesions, and lysis of uterine septa.

✖ The larger resectoscopes are better suited for resection of submucosal myomas and large polyps.

✖ The rotary/twist lock design can unlock while rotating the resectoscope during surgery. The snap-in systems can unlock when moving the resectoscope within the cavity or when removing it from the uterine cavity.

✖ There are four basic designs of resectoscopic electrodes: the (a) loop, (b) bar/barrel, (c) ball, and (d) point or knife-like tip.

✖ Telescopes are available with a viewing angle of 0°, 5°, 12°, 15°, 25°, or 30°. No single angle of vision is best for resectoscopy.

✖ Low viscosity distention media can be delivered using gravity, pumps (Zimmer CDIS, Hamou Hysteromat, and Staflo), or pressure cuffs.

✖ Intrauterine pressure should not exceed 80 mmHg.

✖ Single-chip cameras will generate 300–550 lines of resolution compared with 600–800 lines of resolution generated by three-chip cameras.

✖ Three-chip cameras have increased color separation, resolution, and S/N ratios compared to single-chip camera systems but are almost twice the cost.

✖ Differences in single-chip camera systems include the camera head and telescopic optics; the color reproduction, tone, and tints are essentially the same.

✖ Features to look for with any camera include a small, lightweight camera head with focusing ring and zoom feature (usually 25–40 mm) and a camera system that has automatic adjustments for its various features (gain control, brightness control, color adjustment, and white balance).

✖ Arrangement of equipment should be part of the planning before procedures begin. Placement of the video camera cable, light source cable, electrosurgical cable, and distention media input and output tubing need to be considered.

✖ A clear and unobstructed view of the video monitor that does not cause the surgeon's neck to strain is essential.

✖ Either the circulating nurse or anesthesiologist should be assigned to monitor input/output prior to starting the surgery.

> ✘   The surgeon should have a working knowledge of the video equipment. A complete understanding of how to put together the resectoscope and connect the electrodes and cables is essential for hassle-free surgery.
>
> ✘   If you do not understand your equipment you will one day have to explain to your patient that you had to cancel or could not complete her surgery because of technical difficulties (your usual operating room staff called in sick!).

REFERENCES

1. Neuwirth RS. A new technique for and additional experience with hysteroscopic resection of submucous fibroids. Am J Obstet Gynecol 1978;131:91–94.
2. Haning RV, Harkins, PG, Uehling DT. Preservation of fertility by transcervical resection of a benign mesodermal uterine tumor with a resectoscope and glycine distending medium. Fertil Steril 1980;33: 209–210.
3. DeCherney AH, Polan ML. Hysteroscopic management of intrauterine lesion and intractable uterine bleeding. Obstet Gynecol 1983;61: 392–397.
4. DeCherney AH, Russell JB, Graebe RA, Polan ML. Resectoscopic management of mullerian fusion defects. Fertil Steril 1986;45:726–728.
5. Soderstrom RM. Electricity inside the uterus. Clinical Obstet Gynecol 1992;35(2):262–269.
6. Siegler AM, Valle RF, Lindemann HJ, Mencaglia L. Therapeutic hysteroscopy indications and techniques. St. Louis: CV Mosby, 1990:10–35.
7. Loffer FD. Laser ablation of the endometrium. Obstet Gynecol Clin N Am 1988;15:77–89.
8. Indman PD. Instruments and video cameras for operative hysteroscopy. Clinical Obstet Gynecol 1992;35(20):211–224.

3

The Tissue Effects of Radiofrequency Electrosurgical Currents

Robert D. Tucker

onopolar electrosurgery utilizes alternating radiofrequency (RF) currents to cut and coagulate tissue. Current flows from the electrosurgery generator to the active electrode, to the surgical site tissue, and through the patient's body and is collected at the return electrode or "ground pad"; the circuit is then complete as the current is returned to the generator. In electrosurgery, the active electrode does not heat, but, rather, the tissue heats as it resists the flow of the RF alternating current. Thus, electrosurgical currents accomplish surgical action of cutting and coagulating by heat. This effect is different from true electrocautery, in which electrical currents are used to heat a wire and the hot wire coagulates tissue. Unlike electrosurgery, electrocautery cannot cut tissue or work in a fluid medium.

Electrosurgery began in 1891, when French physicist d'Arsonval discovered that alternating currents at frequencies of 2,000 cycles per second to 2 million cycles per second (2 kHz to 2 MHz, where Hertz or Hz equals cycles per second) when applied to living tissue caused heating without muscle or nerve stimulation (1). By 1910, the American surgeon, William Clark, routinely used electrosurgical coagulation to remove benign and malignant tumors of the head, neck, breast, and cervix (2). In the same year, Edwin Beer utilized radiofrequency alternating current to endoscopically remove bladder tumors and growths at the bladder neck (3). In the mid 1920s, many different electrosurgical machines became commercially available in Europe and the United States. However, it was not until William Bovie, a Harvard physicist, collaborated with Harvey Cushing, the Chief of Surgery at Peter Brent Brigham Hospital, that a machine capable of cutting and coagulating tissue became generally accepted by surgeons (4,5).

Radiofrequency electrosurgery has become commonplace in modern medicine. It has been estimated that 60–80% of all surgical procedures employ electrosurgery. Recent procedural developments in endoscopy and laparoscopy have also led to an increased utilization of electrosurgery. Technological advances have been made that have increased the safety of electrosurgical procedures, e.g., return electrode monitoring for open surgical procedures (6), active electrode shielding and monitoring for monopolar laparoscopic procedures (7), and bipolar electrodes (8).

However, even with a century of scientific and clinical experience with RF electrosurgery, little has been written about the evaluation of the tissue effects of RF currents. This chapter will discuss the biophysics of electrosurgery current flow and its interaction with tissue and then describe the various histological effects.

BIOPHYSICS OF ELECTROSURGERY

Electrosurgical generators supply electrons at a variable voltage. The flow of electrons per second is termed current and is measured in amperes. Voltage, measured in volts, is the amount of force available to push electrons through wire or tissue. As current flows through tissue, the tissue resists the flow; this resistance, measured in ohms (Ω), creates heat, which, in turn, causes desiccation or cutting action.

The amount of tissue heating is proportional to *current (I)* squared, times the *tissue resistance (R)*, or $I^2 \times R = P$. This formula defines the *power (P) delivered to the tissue* and is measured in watts. It is easily seen that for a specific amount of tissue and a given current flow, low resistance tissue will produce less power and, therefore, less heat than high resistance tissue. The resistance of tissue varies dramatically from a low of 30 Ω/cm for blood to high values of 1,000 Ω/cm for fat. Intermediate tissue resistances of 300 to 400 Ω/cm are seen for muscle while liver and bowel present with slightly lower values of 100 to 200 Ω/cm. Coagulated or desiccated tissue will produce resistances from 1,500 to 3,000 Ω/cm. These values are approximate and vary with the saline content of the tissue.

The power formula should, however, be modified to account for another important electrosurgical variable. If the current flow is concentrated in a small area, such as a needle active electrode, the heating effect is typically high, thus producing cutting action. However, if this same current is spread over a large area, such as the return electrode or ground pad, there is virtually no heating. Therefore, the current delivered to a cross–sectional area (A) or the current density (I/A) must be considered in analyzing heat production. This added variable yields a modified power formula of $P = (I/A)^2 \times R$. The effect is easily seen in routine surgery. At a given generator setting, if the current passes through a small appendix–like piece of material, such as an adhesion, the tissue heats and the current flow can create heat damage at a site many centimeters distal to the surgery (9). However, if this same current is applied to a larger area, such as the surface of a large muscle or the bowel, the current effects are seen only several millimeters from the site of surgery. In the latter case, the current spreads over a large area of tissue creating low current densities and, therefore, low heat while the current confined to flow in the adhesion produces a high current density and, therefore, a high temperature.

In determining the extent of tissue damage, the application time must be considered. For example, 50 watts of power applied by contact desiccation for five seconds will produce considerable tissue destruction; however, the same power applied for only one second will produce significantly less tissue necrosis. The variable, which relates to the amount of tissue destruction, is, therefore, the *power* times the *application time (t)* or $P \times t$; this variable is termed the *energy (E = P × t)* and is measured in joules. While energy values correlate with tissue volume necrosis (10), the method of power delivery must be considered, i.e., cut, coagulate, or fulgurate, as well as the time course of power delivery. The time course effect is obvious. For example, 50 W delivered for two seconds produces 100 J of energy; however, 1 W delivered for 100 seconds also produces 100 J, but typically without any tissue effect.

The generator waveform also effects tissue heating. The typical cut waveform is a continuous sine wave that alternates from positive to negative voltage at a frequency of 400 kHz to 3 MHz. The continuous output has the potential to produce high heat and, thus, a cutting action. Coagulation waveforms typically consist of a burst of sine waves with no output between bursts. In these waveforms, the generator delivers current less than twenty-five percent of the time. As a result of these intermittent bursts, the heat is significantly less, leading to tissue desiccation rather than cutting action. Fulguration or spray coagulation is another mode of coagulation waveform. In this mode, the active electrode does not touch the tissue; rather, the high voltage output, up to 10,000 volts, causes breakdown of air into ions and sparking from electrode to tissue. The utilization of this high voltage, low current mode of operation leads to a very thin layer of tissue necrosis and little depth of thermal penetration. The terms *cut waveform* and *coagulation waveform* are somewhat arbitrary. A continuum exists between cut and coagulation waveforms as the cut waveform at lower power settings can cause excellent contact tissue desiccation and a coagulation waveform at high power settings does have cutting action.

TISSUE EFFECTS OF ELECTROSURGERY

The goal of this section is not to turn gynecologists into experts on surgical pathology but rather to provide examples of the effect of RF current on tissue and to guide the gynecologists to aid in the histological evaluation of tissue samples. Most pathologists are unfamiliar with the examination of electrosurgical damage and are reluctant to provide a cause and effect diagnosis. Subtle effects of low temperature (40° to 80°C) are often missed. Therefore, in order to obtain valid information, the gynecologist must be sufficiently familiar with the tissue effects of RF current to provide the necessary input to the pathologist evaluating the samples.

Figures 3-5 to 3-10, 3-12 and 3-13, were sections obtained by contact desiccation on the mucosal surface of pig bladder at 30 W in coagulation mode for three seconds using a Valleylab Force 2™ generator. The samples were then excised immediately and prepared for histologic analysis. Figures 3-11 and 3-3 were obtained utilizing the same procedure on dog stomach mucosa and rabbit uterus, respectively. Figures 3-1 and 3-2 are sections from a human laparoscopic procedure in which the small bowel was desiccated unintentionally; the burn was not excised until one week postsurgery.

Tissue Stains

Unfortunately, there is no one histologic stain that is diagnostic of electrosurgical damage or will allow demarcation of cells that will ultimately undergo necrosis. Therefore, in analyzing electrosurgical damage, it may be necessary to employ multiple stains to determine the extent of damage.

The most commonly and routinely used stain is hematoxylin and eosin (H & E). The stain consists of two parts: hematoxylin, a nuclear stain, and eosin, a negative-charged plasma stain. The hematoxylin stains nuclei blue, while the eosin stains erythrocytes, collagen, and cytoplasm of muscle or epithelial cells varying shades or intensities of pink. Figure 3-1 shows a section of small bowel damaged by electrosurgery and stained with H & E. The stain is readily available in all pathology laboratories. H & E stained slides are excellent for viewing morphology, and most pathologists are comfortable reading H & E stained tissue.

A trichrome stain combines a plasma stain and a connective fiber stain; various trichrome stains are available, including Gomori, Mallory, and Masson. These stains color cell cytoplasm and muscle fibers red, collagen, green or blue, depending upon the specific chemical solution, and nuclei, blue to black. Figure 3-2 shows the same section as Figure 3-1, but stained with trichrome. These three-colored stains give added contrast and, therefore, may make areas of

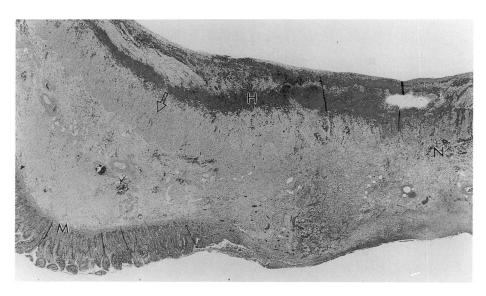

FIGURE 3-1

A section of human ileum that was burned inadvertently on the serosal surface (top of picture). The burn is a full thickness with the necrotic tissue (N) on the right side of the figure. The mucosa (M) on the far left of the figure is normal, but by the middle of the figure, all normal architecture is lost. A large amount of hemorrhage (H) is seen on the entire serosal surface. The muscle fibers facing the mucosa (open arrow) are normal while the muscle near the serosa show thermal damage, including vacuolization.

electrosurgical damage easier to demarcate. As trichrome stains contain a connective tissue stain, they are particularly useful in examining tissues rich in collagen.

Another stain useful in examining electrosurgical thermal damage is picrosirius red. This stain colors collagen and reticulum a deep red, nuclei are colored black, and all other tissue elements are colored bright yellow. As collagen and reticular fibers are strongly anisotropic in longitudinal section, upon viewing with polarized light, the collagen and reticulum fibers show strong birefringence. Denatured collagen and reticulum fibers show little birefringence; this effect is demonstrated in Figure 3-3. The area of rabbit uterus with the electrosurgical thermal damage is shown as a dark red tissue

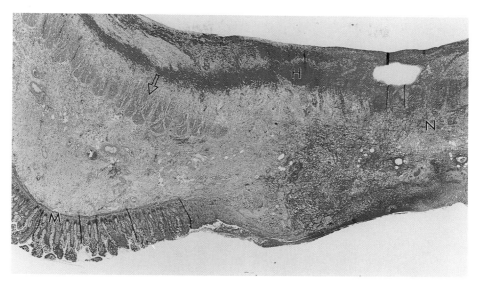

FIGURE 3-2

The adjacent section of tissue as shown in Figure 3-1. This section was stained with Masson trichrome and shows the same histological changes as in Figure 3-1.

with no birefringence while the overlying normal muscle shows strong birefringence at the right side of the picture, which fades toward the left of the figure. The stain is extremely useful at demonstrating thermal damage immediately postelectrosurgical cutting or coagulation. However, damage viewed several days postsurgery may be equivocal. During evaluation, it must be remembered that collagen and reticular fibers are isotropic in cross-section and, therefore, produce little birefringence if cut in that plane.

Histologic View of Electrosurgical Damage

As stated in the previous section, electrosurgical damage is caused by heat. Heating that is rapid and intense, greater than 100°C, will cause the vaporization of intracellular and extracellular fluids, thereby producing a cutting action. Temperatures less than 100°C cause a desiccating or coagulation action. Intracellular and extracellular proteins are irreversibly denatured at temperatures between 80° and 100°C. Tem-

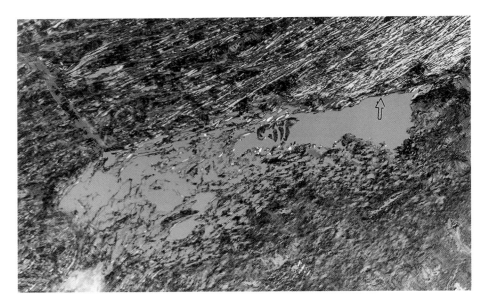

FIGURE 3-3

A section of rabbit fallopian tube contact desiccated for three seconds at 30 W from a Valleylab Force 2 electrosurgical generator. The section is stained with picrosirius red and viewed with polarized light. The dark red tissue in the lower right-hand area is thermally damaged and shows very little birefringence. The tissue overlying the damaged part shows birefringence (open arrow), which fades toward the left of the figure.

peratures between 60° and 80°C will cause reversible damage to some proteins, e.g., the unfolding of collagen chains without destroying the collagen triple helixes. At temperatures of less than 60°C, changes to tissues are more subtle and may be confined to specific cells or specific cellular components.

In an electrosurgical coagulation, the tissue temperature immediately surrounding the active electrode will be the highest; there is a thermal gradient created in which the tissue temperature varies from a high temperature to normal body temperature over a given distance. Figure 3-4 is a diagrammatic representation of the variation of the temperature in tissue over distance for an electrosurgical coagulation. As RF current follows the paths of least resistance and these

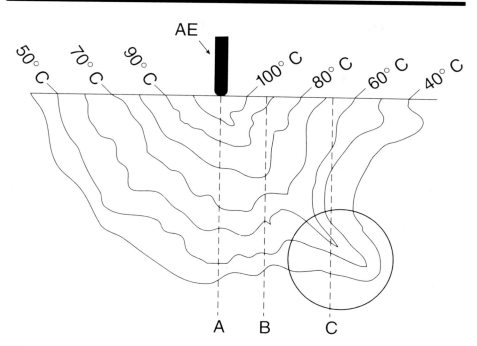

FIGURE 3-4

The figure is a diagrammatic representation of the thermal gradients under-lying an active electrode (AE). The temperatures vary from 100°C immediately under the electrode to 40°C at the outer margin. The isothermal lines will vary dynamically depending upon changes in tissue resistance that effect the heat produced within the tissue. The dotted lines perpendicular to the tissue marked A, B, and C show hypothetical histology sections through the tissue. If a histologic section is taken at section C, the circled area will show a hot spot of over 60°C, which would be surrounded entirely by tissue of much lower temperature and displaying few thermal effects.

paths vary from millisecond to millisecond according to the state of desiccation (or the resistance of the desiccated tissue), the isothermal gradients will not be uniform and will dynamically vary. The thermal gradients may be large as tissue temperatures vary from 100°C to body temperature in a few millimeters. Hot spots distant to the surgical site can be created by the RF current following a low resistance path, such as a blood vessel.

The unpredictable flow of current through low resistance paths is only one uncertainty in the histological evaluation of electro-surgical damage. The plane through which the tissue section is taken also creates variation. Consider the diagrammatic electro-surgical burn in Figure 3-4; if sections are obtained in planes A, B, and C, the histologic analysis will vary greatly. The damage will be easily visible in sections taken through planes A and B as these sections are through high temperature areas in which protein denaturation occurred, while a section taken in plane C will show significantly less thermal effect. However, a systematic analysis would yield thermal damage deep to the electrode tissue contact in the circled area; this "hot spot" would be surrounded by tissue that is close to body temperature and displays little damage.

The effect of variations in temperatures and the differences in stains in analyzing the damage is illustrated in Figures 3-1 and 3-2. These samples were taken from the same tissue block and are adjacent sections. Both sections show the same full-thickness bowel burn without perforation. The mucosal surfaces are toward the bottom of the pictures; the mucosa at the far left of the pictures is normal and progresses toward the right with increasing damage and total loss of normal mucosal architecture by the center of the pictures. Both the H & E and trichrome stains show extensive damage in the right half of the figures; these are areas of high temperature in which the normal architecture is replaced by homogeneous-appearing necrotic tissue. Also in the necrotic area, vacuolization is seen throughout the bowel wall. In lower temperature zones, large amounts of hemorrhage are seen on the serosal surfaces. Thrombi are seen in vessels. At higher power magnification, these vessels show not only red cells but organizing clots with fibrin. In the H & E slide, damage to the muscle layer is difficult to assess; however, the normal muscle architecture is disrupted from the center of Figure 3-1 to the right-hand side of the picture. Analysis of the muscle damage in the trichrome section, Figure 3-2, is significantly easier to assess. In this figure, the muscle fibers adjacent to the serosal surface have been disrupted and large numbers of vacuoles are seen while the muscle nearest to the mucosal surface appears more normal. The fact that the damage on the serosal surface extends further than the mucosal surface and the muscle damage is more extensive on the cells facing the serosal surface confirms that the RF current flow originated on the serosa.

During contact desiccation (i.e., the electrode touching the tissue during activation), temperatures can be quite high and, therefore, tissue destruction considerable. The histological picture underlying the electrode is simple; it consists of complete disruption of the normal tissue architecture and the replacement with homogeneous necrotic tissue. Also seen in areas of intense thermal heat are vacuoles created by the vaporization of fluid and the shrinkage of desiccated tissue. Figure 3-5 shows this effect in pig bladder. Vacu-

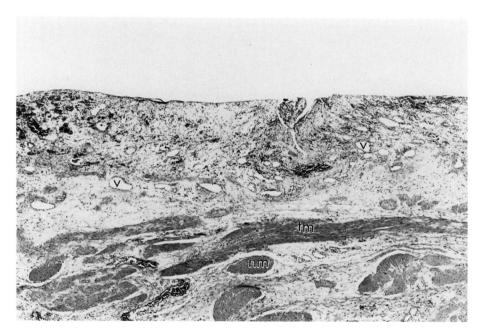

FIGURE 3-5

The mucosal surface of a pig bladder contact desiccated for three seconds at 30 W from a Valleylab Force 2 electrosurgical generator. The entire surface is necrotic with the total loss of normal architecture. Vacuoles (V) are scattered throughout the surface of the figure. Thermally damaged muscle (tm) underlies the necrotic surface and stretches across the entire figure. Underlying the thermally damaged muscle are several normal muscle fibers (nm) (magnification × 10).

The Tissue Effects of Radiofrequency Electrosurgical Currents   37

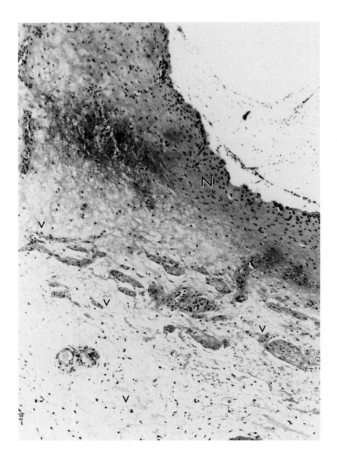

FIGURE 3-6

A section of the mucosal surface of another pig bladder contact desiccated similar to Figure 3-5. The entire surface shows necrotic tissue (N). Underlying the necrotic tissue throughout the section is a fine lacework of small vacuoles (v) created by the vaporization of cellular and extracellular fluids and shrinkage of tissue (magnification × 25).

oles are seen not only near the surface but also deep in the underlying tissue. The entire surface of the section is necrotic, and most of the underlying muscle cells are thermally damaged. Figure 3-6 shows a section from another bladder that demonstrates extensive small vacuoles underlying the necrotic surface. Electrosurgical burn sections, such as this, are easy to diagnose as a result of the large necrotic area and the more subtle tissue changes occurring at the margin of the necrotic area.

High temperature areas denature most proteins and, therefore, produce uniform-appearing necrosis; lower temperatures produce activation of the coagulation cascade, vascular endothelial damage, and thrombi. Even lower temperatures produce thermal damage to vessel walls and bleeding rather than clotting. As a result, slides taken at the periphery of an electrosurgical burn may show considerable hemorrhage. Figure 3-7 demonstrates this effect. At the center, there is a necrotic zone showing little normal architecture. At the periphery

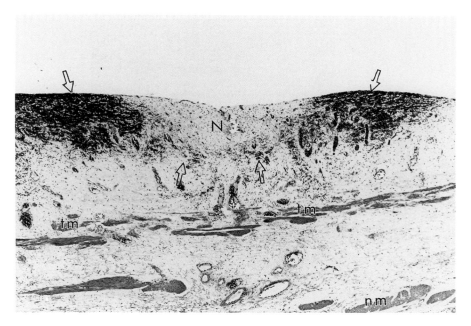

FIGURE 3-7

This section is pig bladder contact desiccated in a similar manner to Figure 3-5. There is a large necrotic area (N) in the center of the figure. Laterally and beneath the necrotic area, there is considerable hemorrhage (open arrows). The muscle cells (tm) spanning the entire figure are elongated and shrunken by thermal damage. Normal muscle (nm) is seen in the bottom right-hand corner (magnification $\times$ 10).

The Tissue Effects of Radiofrequency Electrosurgical Currents   39

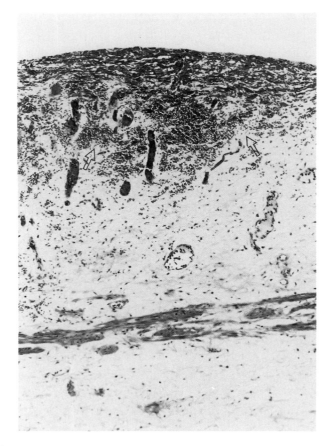

FIGURE 3-8

High magnification of Figure 3-7 showing hemorrhage (open arrows) and underlying thermally damaged muscle (magnification × 25).

of the high temperature zone, there is considerable hemorrhage laterally and some hemorrhage in underlying tissue. Hemorrhage in this section demarcates the necrotic tissue. Much of the underlying muscle layer shows thermal damage. It is impossible to determine if these underlying tissues, which are not overtly necrotic, are viable; however, these areas have sustained sufficient thermal damage that these cells would probably undergo necrosis over time. Only the muscle in the bottom right corner of the figure shows minimal thermal effect. Figure 3-8 shows a higher magnification of the hemorrhage demonstrated in Figure 3-7. The muscle cells underlying the hemorrhage demonstrate considerable thermal damage, including muscle cell elongation and nuclear shape changes. Nuclear changes include elongation, shrinkage, and hyperchromasia.

As discussed earlier, sections taken through low temperature areas may show only subtle electrosurgical damage. As current follows the path of least resistance, blood vessels are particularly susceptible to damage; the damage can occur far from necrotic areas and may be surrounded by totally normal tissue. Figure 3-9, from a

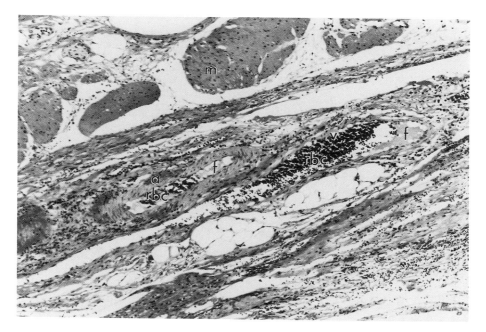

FIGURE 3-9

A section from a pig bladder contact dessicated in a similar manner to Figure 3-5; the section is from a low temperature area removed from mucosal contact desiccation. Muscle cells (m) at the top of the picture are normal. However, beneath the muscle cells, there are two vessels both showing thermal damage. The artery (a) shows nuclear changes in the endothelial cells and a fibrin clot (f) with red blood cells (rbc) occluding the entire lumen. The adjoining vein (v) shows a longitudinal cut with a partially occluding clot with fibrin and red blood cells (magnification × 25).

The Tissue Effects of Radiofrequency Electrosurgical Currents   41

pig bladder, shows an artery and vein surrounded by normal muscle. Within the artery, a clump of red cells is embedded in a fibrin clot; this thrombus has occluded the vessel. This artery endothelium also demonstrates typical nuclear thermal damage. In close approximation is a large vein partially occluded with a fibrin clot. Figure 3-10 shows another pig bladder artery and vein with electrosurgically-caused thrombi. Although connective tissue surrounding the vessels shows heat damage, the muscle immediately adjacent to the vessels demonstrates little thermal effect. Figure 3-11 is a section from a dog stomach taken immediately after the electrocoagulation

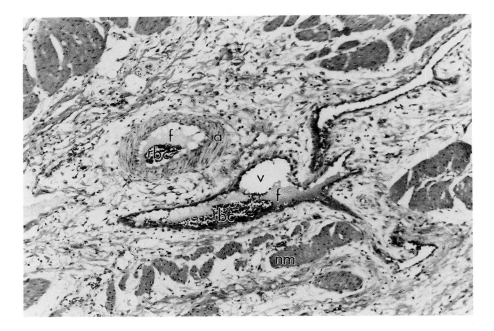

FIGURE 3-10

A section from pig bladder with a contact desiccation on the mucosa created in a manner similar to Figure 3-5. The section shows an artery (a) and vein (v) surrounded by completely normal muscle cells (nm). The artery is occluded by a fibrin clot (f) with embedded red blood cells (rbc). The endothelial cells demonstrate nuclear shape changes from thermal damage. The adjoining vein is also occluded with a large clot (magnification × 25).

42   Gynecologic Resectoscopy

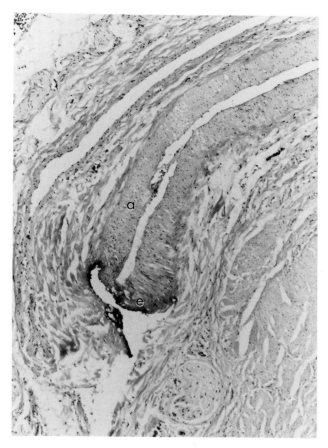

FIGURE 3-11

Section of a dog stomach in which a contact desiccation was performed for three seconds at 30 W with a Valleylab Force 2 electrosurgical generator. The section shows a longitudinal cut of a small artery (a) distant to the mucosal coagulation. The top of the vessel is essentially normal; however, at the center, there is a necrotic area and endothelial damage (e) (magnification × 10).

on the mucosal surface. The figure shows a large vessel in longitudinal section completely surrounded by normal tissue. The great majority of the vessel is totally normal except for a very small area of heat damage to the endothelium at the center of the figure. Such an effect may have been caused by the narrowing of the vessel, creating

The Tissue Effects of Radiofrequency Electrosurgical Currents   43

an increased resistance and, therefore, a larger power with resulting necrosis.

Another subtle effect often overlooked in assessing electrosurgical damage is cellular nuclear change. As nuclei are particularly susceptible to thermal damage, it is important in assessing the extent of the electrosurgical burn to pay close attention to nuclear changes. Figure 3-12 was taken from an electrosurgical coagulation on the mucosa of a pig bladder. The figure demonstrates two muscle bundles, the lower bundle being normal and the upper bundle showing considerable cellular changes. Comparing the nuclei between bundles, the thermally damaged nuclei are hyperchromic and elongated with

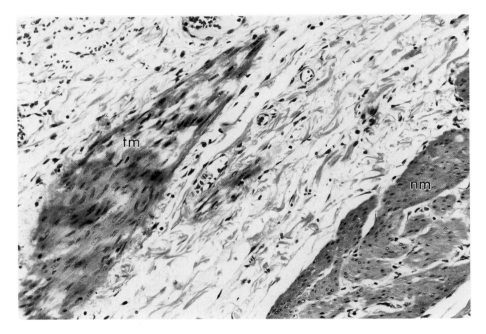

FIGURE 3-12

This is a section from a contact desiccation on pig bladder mucosa performed as described in Figure 3-5. The figure shows two muscle bundles. The lower bundle is normal muscle (nm). The other bundle demonstrates thermally damaged muscle (tm). A comparison of nuclei between bundles shows that the thermally damaged muscle has pyknotic hyperchromic nuclei and few normal nuclei (magnification × 50).

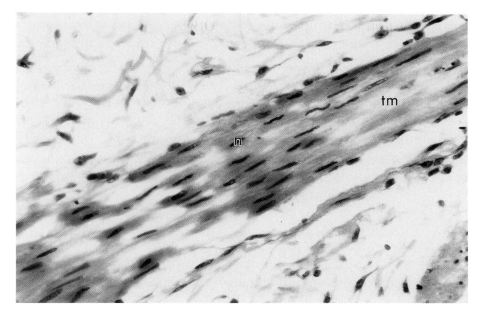

FIGURE 3-13

This is a section from a contact desiccation performed on pig bladder mucosa in a similar manner to Figure 3-5. The figure shows a high magnification of a thermally damaged muscle fiber (tm). The muscle bundle shows the predominance of hyperchromic pyknotic nuclei (n) (magnification × 100).

many showing a twisting confirmation (i.e., pyknotic). Figure 3-13 shows a higher magnification of a muscle bundle; hyperchromic pyknotic nuclei predominate and few normal undamaged nuclei are seen.

CONCLUSIONS

Electrosurgical damage is caused by tissue resisting the flow of RF current, creating heat, and thus, the surgical effect of cutting or desiccating. Tissue damage is related to the energy (or power × time) delivered to the tissue. However, other variables, such as current density and waveform, must also be considered.

The Tissue Effects of Radiofrequency Electrosurgical Currents   45

Tissue damage is a continuum of effects ranging from high temperature denaturing of proteins to low temperature changes. The areas of tissue in high temperature zones undergo necrosis and the complete loss of normal architecture with vacuolization. Tissue in lower temperature zones display varied changes, such as hemorrhage, thrombosis, perivascular damage, and pyknotic hyperchromic nuclei. Unfortunately, it is histologically difficult to determine if tissue in low temperature areas would, with time, necrose. No single histological stain is diagnostic of electrosurgical damage, and in difficult cases, multiple stains may need to be employed to determine cause and effect and to demarcate damaged areas.

REFERENCES

1. d'Arsonval A. Action physiologique des courants alternatifs a grand frequence. Arch Physiol Norm Path 1893;5:401–408, 789–790.
2. Clark WL. Oscillatory desiccation in the treatment of accessible malignant growths and minor surgical conditions: a new electrical effect. J Adv Ther 1911;29:169–183.
3. Beer E. Removal of neoplasms of the urinary bladder. A new method employing high frequency (Oudin) currents through a catheterizing cystoscope. JAMA 1910;54:1768–1769.
4. McLean AJ. The Bovie electrosurgical current generator: some underlying principles and results. Arch Surg 1929;18:1863–1873.
5. Cushing H. Electrosurgery as an aid to the removal of intracranial tumors. With a preliminary note on a new surgical-current generator by W.T. Bovie. Surg Gynecol Obstet 1928;47:751–784.
6. Health devices. ECRI 1985;14(4):115–139.
7. Odell RC. Laparoscopic electrosurgery. In: Hunter J, Sackier J, eds. Minimally invasive surgery. New York: McGraw-Hill, 1993:33–42.
8. Tucker RD, Hollenhorst MJ. Bipolar electrosurgical devices. End Surg 1993;1:110–113.
9. Saye WB, Miller W, Hertzmann P. Electrosurgery thermal injury: myth or misconception? Surg Laparosc Endosc 1991;1(4):223–228.
10. Tucker RD, Kramolowsky EV, Bedell E, Platz C. A comparison of urologic application of bipolar versus monopolar five French electrosurgical probes. J Urol 1989;141:662–665.

4

Applied Electrophysics in Resectoscopic Surgery

Richard M. Soderstrom

All methods of endometrial ablation require the delivery of adequate energy to destroy tissue below the basal layer of the endometrium. The uterus, however, is rich with blood vessels that act as efficient radiators by rapidly removing the intracellular temperature rise. Also, the contour and size of the endometrial cavity will vary from one patient to another. When electrical energy is used to accomplish the task of endometrial ablation, an array of variables, some in the control of the surgeon and some controlled by the physiology, tissue response, and anatomic variation, will dictate the outcome.

Either the resectoscope loop, or roller ball, or both may be used to destroy enough tissue to reduce or eliminate the ability for endometrial regeneration. A roller bar or barrel is also available. Recent experience with a "fat" loop for coagulation shows promise and is before the FDA in review. The endometrial lining, by its own thickness and natural resistance to the flow of electrical energy, can hinder the transfer of enough energy to destroy the basal layers. Medications that reduce the thickness of the endometrium, e.g., GnRH agonists, have been given to the patient several weeks prior to the ablation procedure (see Chapter 7) (1,2). When the clinical situation does not allow for such endometrial preparation, many have used the resecting loop to "shave" the endometrium down to or including the basal layer (see Chapter 12).

At present, there are more theories about which approach gives the best results than there are good outcome statistics (3,4). As one questions the best approach to delivering electrosurgical energy in ablation procedures, the basics of electricity and the variables that must come together to create heat must be understood and appreciated. In the past, surgeons learned electrosurgical technique without any understanding of what was happening at the time of the surgery or the tissue effect after injury occurred. To use the visual endpoint of electrosurgery is far from accurate as to the final outcome. Thus, the principles of electrophysics, as they are applied to endometrial ablation, must be understood by the contemporary gynecologist.

BASIC ELECTRICITY

Electrons are particles of energy that, when pushed (or passed) through human tissue, create heat. This effect may be used to allow cutting or coagulation. Voltage is the pressure force required to push electrons. The standard unit of measure of this "electrical" pressure is one *volt*. Thus, if we draw the analogy of electricity to water, an electron would be analogous to a molecule of water and voltage would be analogous to water pressure.

Whereas volume of water may be measured in cubic centimeters, the volume of electrons is measured in coulombs. If we push a volume of water through a conduit at a given pressure over a specific period, we create *current*. In electricity, current (measured in amperes or coulombs per second) means the passage of a given quantity of electrons through an area over a given period. With either water or electricity, as resistance increases, the flow of current decreases (given constant pressure or voltage). The difficulty of pushing the electrons through tissue or other material can be defined as resistance, measured in *ohms*.

As a last definition, electrical power (measured in *watts*) is the energy produced. The electrical power may be defined as *pressure*

× *current,* or *volts* × *current,* or *volts* × *electron flow per second.* The total energy consumed over a period of time is measured in joules (Table 4-1).

FUNDAMENTALS OF ELECTROSURGERY

Manipulating electrons through living tissue with enough current concentration to create heat and, if desired, tissue destruction, is called *electrosurgery.* Electrogenerators or electrosurgical units are machines that produce an alternating current of electricity at a frequency of 500,000 to 3 million cycles per second, which will not stimulate muscle activity. Whereas direct current flows in one direction only, alternating current flows to and fro, first increasing to a maximum in one direction and then increasing to a maximum in the other direction. This "sinusoidal waveform" can be interrupted or varied, resulting in different surgical effects.

The waveform of alternating current has a negative and a positive excursion or peak. The measurement from 0 polarity to positive or negative polarity is called the *peak voltage* of the waveform (the relationship is the same for peak current). The measurement

TABLE 4-1

Electrophysics Definitions Equated to a Hydraulic Analog

ELECTRICAL CONCEPT	ELECTRICAL UNIT	EQUATIONS	HYDRAULIC ANALOG
Energy	Joule	-----	Energy
Charge	Coulomb (6.3×10^{18} electrons)	-----	Volume (Mass)
Power	Watt	Joules/second	Power
Voltage	Volt	Joules/Coulomb	Pressure Difference
Current	Ampere	Coulombs/second	Flow
Impedence	Ohm	Volts/Ampere	Resistance

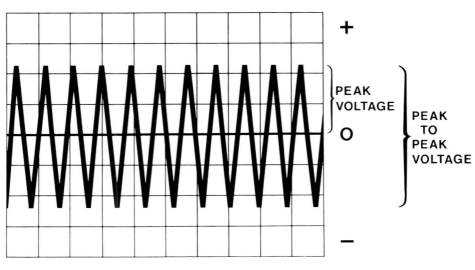

Undamped Waves

FIGURE 4-1

A pure cutting waveform (CUT).

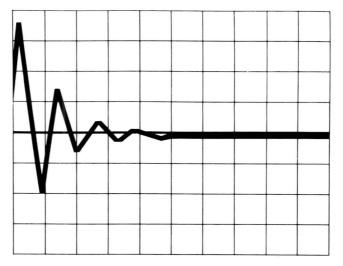

Damped Waves

FIGURE 4-2

A coagulating (COAG) waveform.

from plus peak to negative peak, which is twice peak voltage, is called *peak-to-peak voltage*. A simple sinusoidal, undamped or non-modulated waveform is generally produced by continuous energy and is called a *pure cutting waveform* (CUT) (Figure 4-1). An output waveform that is interrupted or varied (modulated or damped) is called a *coagulating* (COAG) *waveform* (Figure 4-2).

Because of this continuous flow, the peak voltage need not be as high as with the damped waveform to create the same wattage. At the same level, however, when a coagulation effect must be enhanced, the damped waveform is preferable; bursts of damped waveforms are pushed through the tissue. For an instant, with the damped waveform, high voltage may be present within the electrical circuit. A combination of undamped and damped waveforms is called a *blended current* (Figure 4-3).

As electrons, pushed with a given voltage, are concentrated in one specific location, heat within the tissue increases rapidly. This concentration phenomenon is defined as *current density*. The diathermy generator, an example of equipment using this principle, is familiar to most physicians. Here, electrons are passed through the

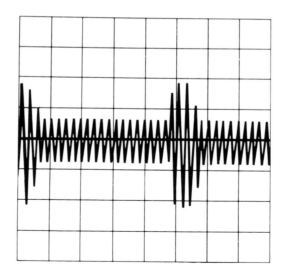

FIGURE 4-3

"Combined" or blended waves giving cutting-coagulation effect.

body by applying two large metal conductors or plates on opposite sides of the body part to be heated. The electrons are pushed through the plate, called the *active electrode*. Electrons are received on the other plate, the *return electrode* or *ground plate,* after they leave the body. Once the electrons enter the body (*conductor*), they are dispersed through the tissue, toward the pathway of least resistance, to the return electrode. Because current is dispersed over the entire surface area of both plates, the heat generated is of low intensity. If either plate is markedly reduced in size, however, current density (and thus heat) is increased accordingly.

Thus, a small active electrode can create a burn where the electrons enter the body. Also, the electrons that leave the body through a small return electrode can produce another burn.

Electrons flow through the path of least resistance. If tissue resistance is high but the corresponding voltage pressure low, the current may cease to flow or may search out alternate pathways with lower resistance. When the voltage is increased, the electrons have more "push" to find an alternate pathway. Such alternate pathways could be through a vital structure where the current might be condensed or where it might lead to an alternate return electrode (i.e., cardiac monitor electrode). Therefore, one should use the lowest voltage necessary to accomplish a given job and be sure that the dispersive electrode is in good contact with the patient and broad enough to reduce current density far below the level of tissue destruction. Isolated ground circuitry systems are desirable, as is a return electrode sentinel system, should an ineffective or incomplete return path be present.

Because operative endoscopy is remote control surgery, it is important that unexpected movements of the electrode do not occur. By reducing peak voltage, you reduce the chance of electrons jumping or sparking to nearby structures. An 8,000-volt pressure can push electrons three millimeters through room air under certain atmospheric conditions. Though many modern generators have a maximum peak voltage of 6,000, most of the time they are used in the 1,000 to 3,000 range.

BIOLOGICAL BEHAVIOR OF ELECTROSURGERY

As mentioned, at the end of an electrode, the performance depends on the shape and size of the electrode, the frequency and wave modulation, the peak voltage, and the current coupled against output impedance. The tissue may be cut in a smooth, deliberate fashion without arching, or it can be burned and charred. This great variation of tissue effects is frequently ignored or misunderstood, which is why some surgeons claim that the laser provides better control of the energy needs and provides better wound healing.

Electrocoagulation may be carried out in many different forms—from slow, delicate contact coagulation (*desiccation*) to the charring effects of the spray coagulation mode (*fulguration*), at times leading to carbonization. The temperature differences may vary between 100°C to over 500°C.

The essential characteristic of CUT waveforms is that they are continuous sinewaves. That is, if the voltage output of the generator is plotted over time, a pure CUT waveform is a continuous sinewave alternating from positive to negative at the operating frequency of the generator, 500 to 3,000 kHz.

The COAG waveform consists of short bursts of radio frequency sinewaves. With the sinewave frequency of 500 kHz, the COAG bursts occur 31,250 times/second. The important feature of the COAG waveform is the pause between each burst. If a COAG waveform had the same peak voltage as a CUT waveform, the average power delivered (heat per second) would be less because the COAG is turned off most of the time (Figure 4-4).

A COAG waveform with the same *average* voltage (RMS voltage) as the CUT waveform could deliver the same heat per second. Because the COAG is turned off most of the time, it can only produce the same RMS voltage as the CUT by having large peak voltages and currents during the periods when the generator is on (Figure 4-5).

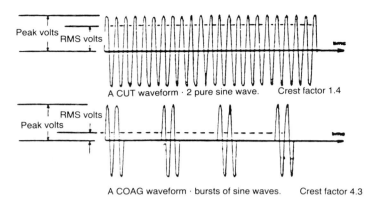

A CUT waveform · 2 pure sine wave.   Crest factor 1.4

A COAG waveform · bursts of sine waves.   Crest factor 4.3

FIGURE 4-4

Equal peak voltage waveforms. The peak voltage is the same in both of these waveforms, but the power is about one-third in the COAG waveform.

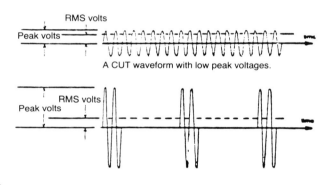

A CUT waveform with low peak voltages.

FIGURE 4-5

Equal power waveforms. A COAG waveform with equal power (energy per second) to the above CUT waveform. Note that the COAG peak voltage is about three times higher in this example. Note also that the root mean square voltages are equal.

A good COAG waveform can spark to tissue without significant cutting effect because the heat is more widely dispersed by the long sparks and because the heating effect is intermittent. The temperature of the water in the cells does not get high enough to flash into steam. In this way, the cells are dehydrated slowly but are not torn apart to form an incision. Because the high peak voltage is a quality of the COAG waveform, it can drive a current through high resistances. In this way, it is possible to fulgurate long after the water is driven out of the tissue and actually char it to carbon. *Coagulation* is a general term which includes both desiccation and fulguration.

Fulguration can be contrasted with desiccation in several ways. First, sparking to tissue with any practical fulguration generator always produces necrosis anywhere the sparks land. This is not surprising considering each cycle of voltage produces a new spark, and each spark has an extremely high current density. In desiccation, the current is no more concentrated than the area of contact between the electrode and the tissue (Figure 4-6).

As a result, desiccation may or may not produce necrosis, depending on the current density. For a given level of current flow, fulguration is always more efficient at producing necrosis. However, the depth of tissue injury is quite superficial compared to contact dessication because with fulguration the sparks jump from one spot to another in a random fashion, thus the energy is "sprayed" rather than concentrated (Figure 4-7). In general, fulguration requires only one-fifth the average current flow of desiccation.

For example, if a roller ball electrode is pressed against moist

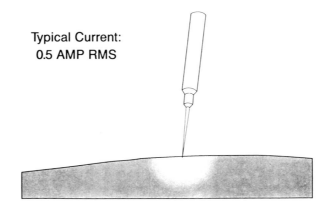

Typical Current:
0.5 AMP RMS

FIGURE 4-6

Desiccation.

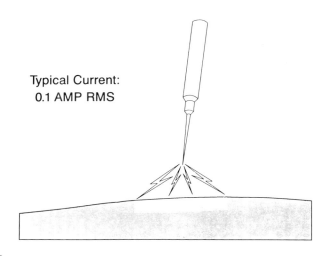

Typical Current:
0.1 AMP RMS

FIGURE 4-7

Fulguration.

tissue, the electrode will begin in the desiccation mode, regardless of the waveform. The initial tissue resistance is quite low and the resulting current will be high, typically 0.5 to 0.8 A RMS. As the tissue dries out, its resistance rises until the electrical contact is broken. Since moist tissue is no longer touching the electrode, sparks will jump to the nearest areas of moist tissue in the fulguration mode, as long as the voltage is high enough to make a spark. Eventually, the resistance of desiccated tissue will stop the flow of electrons limiting the depth of coagulation.

Electrosurgical electrodes can be sculptured to perform certain tasks. A microneedle, a knife, a wire loop, or even a scissor can be shaped and sized to a specific duty. When the waveform variable is added, "cutters" can be made to coagulate and "coagulators" can be made to cut. The faster an electrode passes over or through tissue, the less the coagulation effect leading to more cutting (Figure 4-8). The more broad the electrode, the less cutting and more coagulation effect (Figure 4-9). Interwoven into these acts are the output intensity and output impedance characteristics of the different electrosurgical generators.

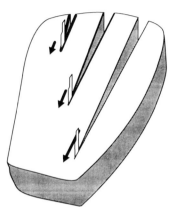

FIGURE 4-8

Influence of the speed of incision on the degree of coagulation.

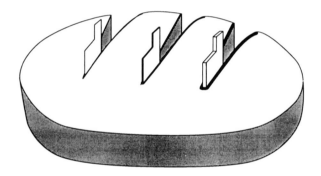

FIGURE 4-9

Influence of the shape of the electrode on the degree of coagulation.

APPLIED ELECTROPHYSICS TO OPERATIVE HYSTEROSCOPY

Endometrial ablation may be performed by shaving the endometrial lining with the loop electrode (see Chapter 12) or desiccating the endometrial lining with the roller ball or bar. A few surgeons shave first and then "paint" the shaved myometrium with the roller electrode. Unfortunately, studies on the tissue effects of different techniques, electrodes, and waveforms are few. Even the pressure applied to the endometrial surface will change the current (power) density; the more pressure, the broader the contact surface of the electrode will be, creating a decreased current density. The speed of movement of the electrode over the endometrium is unique to each surgeon (another variable). Only the outcome statistics can be evaluated reasonably. Some use a coagulation-only waveform at a low wattage of 30; others report success with a pure cutting waveform at 100 W.

My personal preference is to shave the endometrium first. I use a pure undamped waveform and drag the wire loop in a slow, deliberate motion to four millimeters deep through the tissue so there is some coagulation effect in addition to cutting properties. By using the cutting waveform, bubble formation on the anterior surface of the endometrial cavity is less than in the coagulation mode. I do not shave the cavity's lateral sulcus near the uterine vessels.

During the "painting" phase, I continue to use an undamped waveform with a light contact of the roller electrode set at 100 W. If the roller electrode is a bar or barrel, I will either slow up the rolling motion or increase the power output because the electrode current density is lower. At the end of the ablation procedure, I will switch to a coagulation waveform at 75 W. With the increased peak voltage of this waveform, skip areas will be "sought out" by the electrons under higher pressure, assuring complete surface coagulation.

On seven hysterectomy specimens, histologic studies performed several months after the ablation procedure demonstrated a complete absence of the endometrial lining, replaced by cuboidal cells, and a coagulation depth into the myometrium of 3 to 5 mm. Still, the total amenorrhea rate using this technique in 100 cases has been only 60%. Thirty-five percent of the patients have tolerable oligomenorrhea, the failure rate being 5%. These statistics do not differ from those of surgeons who use lower power settings, one electrode and either blended or coagulation waveforms (5,6,7).

HAZARDS

Two-thirds of electrical accidents during operative hysteroscopy occur at the return electrode site. As with all surgical procedures where electrosurgical generators are used, the operating room staff need to possess the proper techniques for return electrode application. Both the staff and surgeon should have some familiarity with the instruction manual supplied with the generators as with lasers.

To date, true electrical injuries within the uterus have been few and have been associated with inadvertent perforation, partial or incomplete. Though some have worried about sparking or arching through the uterine wall to adjacent structures, the physics of fulguration make this unlikely. Because a nonelectrolytic solution is used for distention, fluid overload has occurred (see Chapter 14).

OTHER STUDIES

Several in vitro studies have tried to answer the questions surrounding the best power settings and choice of waveform to reach consistent results. Unfortunately, without an intact circulation, such a model cannot represent a simile of the in situ uterus. One study found more microscopic heat effect when the power was increased in the coagulation mode of the generator, although they only evaluated the tissue effect using a hematoxylin and eosin (H & E) tissue stain, which does not take into account the death of respiratory enzymes in those cells adjacent to the obvious areas of destruction (8). Another study, using a similar in vitro model, showed a slight linear difference in tissue effect when the power applied was at equal levels. When the desiccation/cut waveform was compared to the fulguration/coagulation waveform, the former appeared to achieve a more consistent tissue effect (9). In this study, a phosphatase stain used to highlight those cells whose respiratory enzymes had been destroyed was inclusive. This is in contrast with similar studies, yet to be published, where the phosphatase stain clearly revealed enzyme deficiency several millimeters below the layer of obvious cellular destruction (Soderstrom RM, Vancaillie TG. Personal communication, January 1994).

In the H & E study, the in vitro model was a bivalved uterus in which the active electrode was applied in an open air environment. In the second study using hematoxylin and eosin plus the phosphatase stain, the same model was used but placed in a saline bath. Since saline is a good conductor of electricity, a reduction in current density may have occurred. In the unpublished study, the in vitro model was an intact, extirpated uterus where the electrode roller ball was applied through the cervix using a continuous flow resectoscope and glycine as a distending medium.

Until a series of in vitro studies using both microscopic stains and respiratory enzyme evaluation are completed, clinical outcome events will be our best method of choosing the amount of joules needed to complete the task. Even then, the size/shape and speed of application of the ablation electrode will be hard to set in a controlled manner.

SUMMARY

Although electrosurgery has been practiced by surgeons for decades, few have received formal training in its proper uses. The erroneous belief that electrosurgery techniques increase scar formation or impair healing processes has led surgeons to other methods to deliver energy to the living cell. At the cellular level, a watt is a watt and is independent of its power source—knowing how to calculate and administer that energy is the challenge. Laser technology has forced bioelectrical engineers to develop improved electrogenerators and accessories that are easier to understand and control. The use of digital reader boards, displayed in watts rather than an arbitrary dial setting, is one example. A good electrosurgical system, with proper accessory electrodes, is only 10% of the cost of the average laser. For hysteroscopic resectoscopy procedures, a thorough knowledge and appreciation of the physics of electrosurgery is a basic requirement.

The most common use of electrical surgery in intrauterine surgery is for endometrial ablation. The principles that apply to this use can be extrapolated to other uses, such as septum excision and fibroid resection.

REFERENCES

1. Brooks PG, Serden SP, Davos I. Hormonal inhibition of the endometrium for resectoscopic endometrial ablation. Am J Obstet Gynecol 1991;164:1601–1608.
2. Brooks PG, Serden SP. Preparation of endometrium for ablation with a single dose of leuprolide acetate depot. J Reprod Med 1991;36:477–482.
3. Indman P, Soderstrom R. Depth of endometrial coagulation with the urologic resectoscope. J Reprod Med 1990;35:633–635.
4. Indman P, Brown W. Uterine surface changes caused by electrosurgical endometrial coagulation. J Reprod Med 1992;37:667–670.
5. Vancaillie TG. Electrocoagulation of the endometrium with the ball-end resectoscope ("rollerball"). Obstet Gynecol 1990;76:425–427.
6. Townsend DE, Richart RM, Paskowitz PA, Woolfork RE. "Rollerball" coagulation of the endometrium. Obstet Gynecol 1989;74:310–331.
7. DeCherney AH, Diamond MD, Lavy G, Polan ML. Endometrial ablation for intractable uterine bleeding: hysteroscopic resection. Obstet Gynecol 1987;70:668–670.
8. Letterie GS, Hibbert ML, Britton BA. Endometrial histology after electrocoagulation using different power settings. Fertil Steril 1993;60:647–651.
9. Onbargi LC, Hayden R, Valle RF, Del Priore G. Effects of power and electrical current density variations in an in vitro endometrial ablation model. Obstet Gynecol 1993;82:912–918.

5

Distention Media

Eric J. Bieber

T he effective use of distending media is one of the most important aspects for improving visualization and decreasing hysteroscopic complications. While urologists have contended with the difficulties of distention and media choice for resectoscopy over the last five or six decades, gynecologists have only recently retraced their steps. This chapter describes all of the media commonly used for hysteroscopic surgery and focuses on those solutions that have the greatest utility in operative and electrosurgical hysteroscopy.

THE DIFFICULTY WITH DISTENTION

While many parallels exist between urologic cystourethroscopy/ resectoscopy and gynecologic hysteroscopy, significant differences are present. The cervix is not easily dilated and represents a barrier to surgery. The uterus is significantly more muscular, and, thus, greater pressure (as compared to the bladder) is necessary to allow separation of the endometrial walls. This separation allows the potential space of the uterus to become a true space in which surgery may be effectively performed. Unfortunately, because of the vascular nature of the uterus overdistention may not improve visualization past a certain threshold but may predispose the patient to a greater risk of fluid intravasation (Figure 5-1). Depending on the indication for surgery and type of instrumentation to be used, one medium may be more appropriate than another. A list of media commonly used in hysteroscopy is found in Table 5-1. Several factors are important in selecting a medium, including the type of surgery to be performed, amount of bleeding anticipated at the time of surgery, and the need for electrosurgery. The optimal medium would have clear visibility with a refractive index of 1.00, be isotonic, allow easy cleansing of instruments used during surgery, and have minimal impact on plasma, extracellular and intracellular fluid volumes (Table 5-2). In addition, cost per liter of solution differs markedly between each fluid (Table 5-3). Unfortunately, this perfect medium does not exist, and as surgeons, we must know the benefits, risks, and limitations of multiple media to choose the most appropriate for a given surgery.

TABLE 5-1

Media Commonly Used for Hysteroscopy

Low Viscosity Media	
Electrolyte Containing	
LR	
0.45 / 0.9 NS	
Nonelectrolyte Containing	
Glycine	(1.5%)
Sorbitol	(3%)
Mannitol	(5%)
Cytal (sorbitol/mannitol)	(3.2%)
D_5W	
High Viscosity Media	
Hyskon	
Gas Media	
Carbon Dioxide	

LR = Lactated Ringer's
NS = normal saline

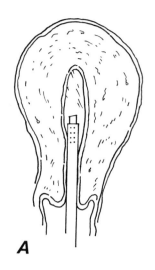
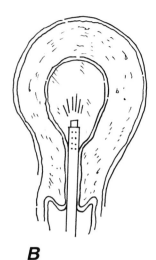

A

B

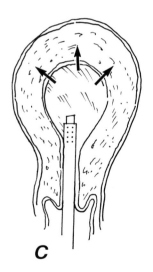

C

FIGURE 5-1

(A) Underdistention of the uterine cavity resulting in inadequate separation of the walls and decreased visualization; (B) adequate distention with excellent visualization; (C) increased intrauterine pressures giving no visual improvement but causing an increase in media intravasation.

TABLE 5-2

Characteristics of an "Ideal" Medium

Isotonic
Clear visibility
Ease of instrument cleaning
Minimal impact on body fluid volumes
Ease of hysteroscopic delivery
Nonhemolytic
Nonconductive

TABLE 5-3

Cost Comparison of Various Media

Solution	Size of Bag	Cost in Dollars Per Unit*
1.5% glycine	5L	19.70
1.5% glycine	3L	12.20
3.0% sorbitol	5L	19.70
3.0% sorbitol	3L	12.20
0.9% NS	1L	3.66
0.9% NS	2L	6.66
0.9% NS	3L	9.75
LR	3L	10.50
LR	5L	17.00
D_5W	1L	6.58

*List prices from Baxter.

TYPES OF DISTENTION MEDIA

Carbon Dioxide (CO_2)

Carbon dioxide is a gas medium with excellent optical properties, and it is relatively easy to use. Its refractive index is 1.00, or essentially equivalent to air. Carbon dioxide has found the greatest utility in diagnostic hysteroscopy, but has limited applicability to operative hysteroscopy or resectoscopy because of the bleeding encountered during these procedures. The low viscosity of CO_2 allows easy flow through the relatively small inflow portals of most hysteroscopes. Unfortunately, this characteristic allows CO_2 to migrate around the hysteroscope and out the cervical os if overdilation has occurred.

Rubin first reported on the use of CO_2 to distend and view the endometrium in patients with infertility (1). He used a modified cystoscope and performed most of these procedures in the office setting. He later reported on the safety of using CO_2 to evaluate tubal patency in over 80,000 patients (2).

While excellent for diagnostic studies, the inability of CO_2 and blood to mix limits its application. The bubbles formed from this interaction can obscure the view and limit what can be successfully performed hysteroscopically.

Although a long safety history exists for CO_2 used hysteroscopically, there are concerns regarding potential problems if inappropriate insufflators are used. Dedicated hysteroscopic CO_2 insufflators have been manufactured for several decades. These insufflators are preset to either limit flow or pressure to below 100 mL/min or 200 mmHg. Generally excellent visualization is possible at pressure settings of 60 to 80 mmHg with an average flow rate of 50 mL/min. Laparoscopic insufflators (even older models) should never be used for hysteroscopy. The flow rates of >1000 mL/min could cause a CO_2 pulmonary embolus. Baggish and Daniel reported on significant complications, including mortalities, from CO_2-cooled Nd-YAG laser tips being used for hysteroscopic ablation (3). These cases demonstrate, in vivo, the risk of CO_2 emboli in high flow systems where tissue disruption allows subsequent emboli formation.

Carbon dioxide remains an excellent medium for diagnostic evaluation. Its value for operative work is limited to simple operative procedures, such as IUD removal, polypectomy, or directed endometrial sampling. There is no role for CO_2 as a medium when using the resectoscope.

Normal Saline, Lactated Ringer's

Normal saline may be the optimal medium for performance of hysteroscopy using the Nd–YAG laser but has no utility when performing electrosurgery with the operative hysteroscope or resectoscope. Like other low viscosity fluids, saline readily mixes with blood. This is an advantage when using a continuous flow instrument or an operative sheath with multiple ports. With these apparatus, the blood and saline mixture may be suctioned until a clear field is obtained. Optical characteristics for saline show a refractive index of 1.37. Although this is slightly different from CO_2, little difference may be appreciated clinically.

The greatest advantage of normal saline is its isotonicity. Attention must still be paid to the amount of intravasation as fluid overload may still occur. However, there is little concern regarding the possibility of hyponatremia should there be excess intravasation.

Lactated Ringer's is also an isotonic solution, but like normal saline, it contains electrolytes and is an unsatisfactory medium for electrosurgery.

Several manufacturers of electrosurgical generators are evaluating systems that would allow concurrent use of electrodes and saline as a distention medium. Presently, if standard electrosurgical generators are used with saline as a distending medium, no significant effect is achieved and the current diffuses in all directions. During a recent endometrial ablation, midway through the case, there was no tissue effect by the ball electrode. The problem was traced to the hanging of a 3-L bag of normal saline instead of 1.5% glycine. On changing back to glycine, the desired electrosurgical effect was reinstated. Fortunately, it is unlikely that a significant current density could be achieved to cause a remote thermal injury in this type of situation.

D₅W or Water

Dextrose 5% in water or water solutions are effective low viscosity solutions. However, they have even greater limitations than normal saline or lactated Ringer's. Although electrolytically non-conductive, both have the disadvantage of causing dilutional hyponatremia. This is especially true for D_5W, which may markedly increase plasma volume, further exacerbating the hyponatremic nature of the solution. Like normal saline, both solutions mix well with blood and, theoretically, may be used in high flow situations.

Water has optical properties that provide excellent visualization. This medium is severely limited in its operative indications by virtue of its ability to cause intravascular hemolysis and subsequent potential for renal damage (4). It is for these reasons that water is not appropriate as a medium choice for hysteroscopy.

Glycine

Glycine is a distention medium commonly used by both gynecologists and urologists. The solution is a low viscosity fluid, composed of a 1.5% mixture of the amino acid and commonly supplied in convenient 3,000 cm³ bags (Figure 5-2). This decreases the need for inconvenient nursing changes of distending media containers. Glycine has been the choice of urologists for decades in performing transurethral resections of the prostate because of its excellent optical properties and lack of electrolytes (5).

Although some authors have referred to glycine as an isotonic fluid, it has an osmolality of only 200 mosm/L and is a hypotonic fluid (6). While posing little risk of intravascular hemolysis, there is a significant risk of volume overload and concurrent hyponatremia should this occur (7).

Glycine metabolism is demonstrated in Figure 5-3. Once glycine has been intravasated, the intravascular half-life is 85 minutes. Following this, the amino acid is broken down to ammonia and

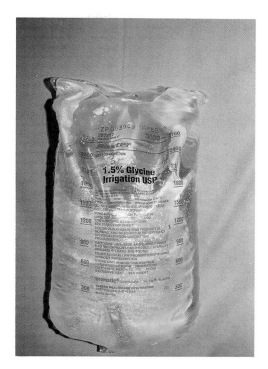

FIGURE 5-2

Large, 3-liter bag of 1.5% glycine.

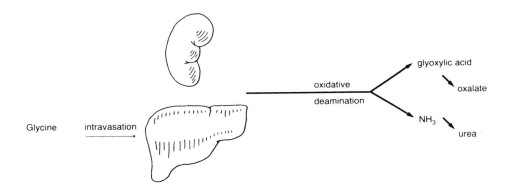

Glycine   intravasation   oxidative deamination

glyoxylic acid → oxalate

NH_3 → urea

FIGURE 5-3

Graphic depiction of glycine's metabolism.

glyoxylic acid via oxidative deamination in the liver and kidney. Ammonia is subsequently excreted as urea, and glyoxylic acid may be further reduced to oxalate.

It is unclear whether patients with underlying renal or hepatic abnormalities may be predisposed to elevated levels of the by-products of glycine metabolism. One report suggested hyperammonemia from excessive glycine metabolism during a transurethral resection of the prostate (TURP) caused clinical toxicity, whereas other reports suggested there is no correlation in these levels even in patients with underlying liver abnormalities (4,8). Oral L-arginine has been suggested as a protective agent, as it promotes ammonia breakdown through the urea cycle (9).

Glycine has been associated with acute, but transient, visual changes. In a small study, four of 18 patients experienced some level of visual alteration (10). It is believed glycine acts as a neuroinhibitory substance at the retina, causing these reversible changes. Although cases of temporary postsurgical blindness have occurred, we know of no report of persistence.

Duffy and colleagues compared electrical parameters of 1.5% glycine, D_5W, distilled water, and deionized water using a resectoscope in an in vitro experiment (11). They found little difference in electrical properties between the four media. Interestingly, they found the addition of blood in varying concentrations resulted in current limiting and eventual electrosurgical generator shutdown (11). They suggest that this situation may occur clinically when the surgeon is operating an electrode in a cavity with excess bleeding, demonstrating the importance of a functioning continuous flow system.

Sorbitol and Mannitol

Sorbitol and sorbitol/mannitol (Cytal-Abbott Laboratories, North Chicago, IL) solutions have also been utilized for years by urologists and are available in large 3,000 cm^3 bags. These solutions have similar problems as glycine in that they are hypotonic and may induce volume overload and hyponatremia if extensive intravasation were to occur. Cytal contains both 2.7% sorbitol and

0.54% mannitol. The mannitol was added to induce diuresis should fluid overload occur. Although anecdotal reports exist regarding the use of these agents during hysteroscopic surgery, there is little information regarding risk and benefit versus other distention agents.

Mannitol and sorbitol have similar structures in that they are both six-carbon molecules (Figure 5-4). However, they are metabolized and act very differently. Sorbitol is broken down to glucose and fructose, whereas little mannitol is metabolized. Because of its short half-life and subsequent renal excretion, mannitol acts effectively as an osmotic diuretic.

Increasing concern has been voiced as the literature becomes replete with reports of fluid overload and hyponatremia. This has focused attention on finding the "best" medium possible. Because of its short half-life and the osmotic diuresis it induces, mannitol may come closest. While low percentage mannitol solutions have an inadequate osmolar concentration, 5% mannitol has been suggested as an ideal medium (6). At this concentration, the solution has an

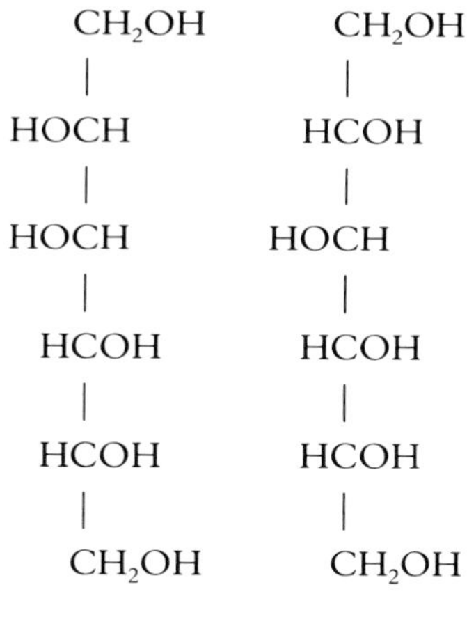

$$
\begin{array}{cc}
CH_2OH & CH_2OH \\
| & | \\
HOCH & HCOH \\
| & | \\
HOCH & HOCH \\
| & | \\
HCOH & HCOH \\
| & | \\
HCOH & HCOH \\
| & | \\
CH_2OH & CH_2OH \\
\\
\text{D-Mannitol} & \text{L-Sorbitol}
\end{array}
$$

FIGURE 5-4

Chemical structure of mannitol and sorbitol, demonstrating marked similarity.

osmolarity of 274 mosm/L, closely approximating the osmolarity of serum (280 mosm/L).

Some writers have voiced concern regarding the "stickiness" of the solution and a potential for carmelization at the electrode. Further evaluations may need to be performed clinically to substantiate mannitol as the preferential medium.

Hyskon

Hyskon is a high viscosity solution composed of dextran 70 (32% W/V) in 10% dextrose (W/V). It contains glucose manufactured into high molecular weight (70 kd) polymers. This solution has been effectively used for hysteroscopy and has also been used as a post-surgical adjuvant to attempt to decrease adhesions. Such a solution was first introduced for endoscopy in 1970 by Edstrom and Fernstrom (12). The solution is highly viscous, clear, and nonconductive since it contains no electrolytes (13). In addition, the solution is poorly miscible with blood and is thus an excellent medium for performing operative hysteroscopy. Similar concerns have been expressed about the use of Hyskon, like mannitol for resectoscopy, in that both solutions may allow for carmelization around the active electrode. A more salient concern may be the inability to have adequate continuous flow given current hysteroscope design. Although the viscous nature of Hyskon reduces the large fluid volumes needed when using low viscosity fluids, it is critical in operative hysteroscopy to have the ability to intermittently remove blood and/or debris from the operative field. It is likely that future instrument modifications will allow the use of resectoscopic electrodes and have multiple ancillary ports for accessory instrumentation or suction devices.

Because of the viscous nature of Hyskon, instruments must be specially cared for following a procedure. I have personally had a hysteroscope ruined because the instrument was not adequately cleaned on procedure completion. The solution will adhere to optical surfaces, valves, and intake and outflow portals. Use of hot water and cleansing solutions obviates these problems.

Another difficulty with Hyskon is the mechanism of delivery. The viscous nature of the solution makes delivery through the rela-

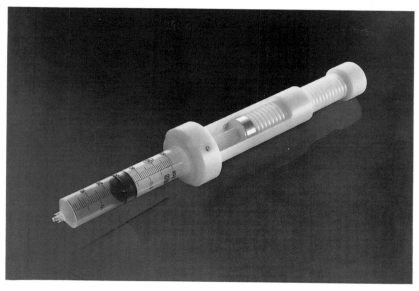

FIGURE 5-5

A hand–held device for delivering Hyskon through hysteroscope channels (Courtesy of Cook OB/GYN).

tively small inflow channels of the hysteroscope somewhat difficult. Several devices for delivery have been created to decrease these difficulties and are further discussed in Chapter 2. A simple hand-held device using Archimedes principle allows easy, effective distention when using Hyskon (Figure 5-5).

COMPLICATIONS FROM DISTENDING MEDIA

While hysteroscopy has a very low rate of significant complications, many are associated with problems of distending media. It should be no surprise that more reports of such complications are being published as more surgeons become familiar with operative hysteroscopic techniques. The previous pages detail the multiplicity of media available to the hysteroscopic surgeon. In the next pages, we will discuss the dynamics of fluid distention, methods for evaluating intravasation, and the differential risks for low and high viscosity media. Methods of avoiding distention media complications and treatment of these complications are described.

DYNAMICS OF UTERINE DISTENTION

Evaluation and surgical treatment within the uterine cavity require adequate distention of the walls to allow panoramic hysteroscopy to be performed. Methods for achieving distention are discussed in Chapter 2. No distention system presently incorporates true monitoring of intrauterine pressure. Adequate uterine distention is usually achieved at 75 mmHg intrauterine pressure, and elevating levels beyond 100 mmHg may increase fluid intravasation risks without beneficial visual improvement. Low viscosity fluid bags attached to a hysteroscope with large-bore urologic tubing will give pressures of 73 mmHg at 1 meter and 110 mmHg at 1.5 meters above the supine patient (14).

When using continuous-flow systems, such as that with a gynecologic resectoscope, one must balance the need to achieve adequate intrauterine pressure with the requirement for outflow suction. Outflow may be obtained by draining (through gravity) into a calibrated canister or into a perineal drape (Figure 5-6), which may then be suctioned into a canister. An alternative would be to directly attach the outflow to a wall suction unit. This allows the surgeon to increase or decrease outflow by manipulation of the outflow valve. The latter method is the author's preference and offers the advantage of the media exiting the resectoscope directly into calibrated canisters. It should be noted that even with this setup, a perineal drape and additional suction is placed in an attempt to account for fluid lost from the hysteroscope and around the cervix. The additional factors that effect intrauterine fluid dynamics include loss of fluid transtubally and fluid loss through intravasation (Figure 5-7). It is this continuously changing surgical need that makes it difficult to develop the perfect automatic device for fluid injection. Such a device

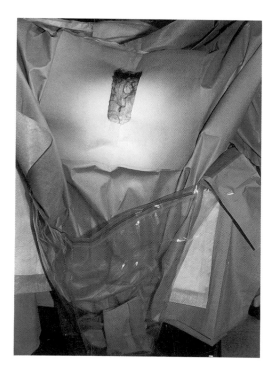

FIGURE 5-6

Perineal pouch for collection of fluid runoff.

would need to monitor intrauterine pressure and make inflow adjustments to maintain this pressure while allowing various levels of outflow just sufficient to keep the field clear and the surgeon happy. In addition, calibration directly from inflow and on the outflow could limit the inherent variation that may exist between 3-L bags of fluid and allow a more accurate assessment of fluid status.

METHODS FOR EVALUATION OF FLUID LOSS

Besides the extraction of fluid via gravity or suction through the outflow channel and loss from around the instrument, media loss may occur partially through ostial/tubal loss, and mainly through

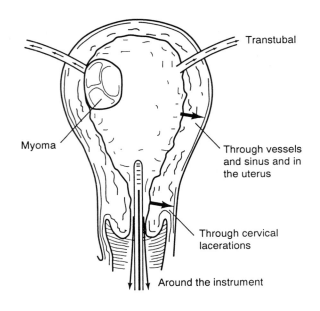

Transtubal

Myoma

Through vessels
and sinus and in
the uterus

Through cervical
lacerations

Around the instrument

FIGURE 5-7

Graphic depiction of where media loss occurs.

intravasation. Intrauterine pressures adequate for visualization (75 to 100 mmHg) will result in little transtubal media passage. Pressures above 100 mmHg are associated with higher levels of transtubal loss. This loss is limited by the closure of the ostium by smooth muscle surrounding the tubal orifice. A similar mechanism is seen during performance of hysterosalpingography, where increased pressure from dye injection causes a contraction of the muscle surrounding the ostium leading to a potential false-positive result of tubal occlusion.

It is not surprising that Baumann and colleagues reported finding glycine in the peritoneal fluid of a patient undergoing transcervical endometrial resection (15). Although certain rationale exist regarding whether tubal occlusion should be performed before or after endometrial ablation, there is no agreement on what effect this has, if any, on the amount of medium intravasation. Magos and colleagues reported a nonstatistically significant decrease in fluid loss if tubal occlusion was performed prior to ablation (16), whereas

Lomano found no difference in absorption of normal saline in patients undergoing Nd–YAG laser ablation who had previously undergone sterilization (17).

It is likely that transtubal medial passage causes increased peritoneal fluid leading to absorption. The clinical significance of this occurrence is mainly that whatever fluid is absorbed by the peritoneum will likely become intravascular and might serve to exacerbate cases of fluid overload. In cases where concurrent laparoscopy is being performed, suction of the fluid may be performed and added to that fluid collected from the hysteroscopic outflow tract.

Most fluid is absorbed via the vascular tree of the uterus. Even at low levels of intrauterine pressure some level of intravasation is difficult to avoid. Although unlikely to be a problem during diagnostic cases, the nature of operative hysteroscopy predisposes to these difficulties. The increased length of time and the dissection of tissue cause endometrial trauma and likely open blood vessels, which under the pressure necessary for adequate visualization, allow intravasation. When one considers the amount of vascularity a leiomyoma may have, it is understandable how myoma shaving would create open channels through which media might flow. It does not take a large surface area to have significant fluid loss as demonstrated by the amount of fluid that may be given through a relatively small 20- or 22-gauge IV catheter when the IV bag has a blood pressure cuff surrounding it.

Multiple factors will ultimately impact on the amount of intravasation, but significant variability will still exist between very similar cases. *It is for this reason that fluid monitoring is essential during all operative hysteroscopic cases.* Additional variables that may lead to increased fluid loss include the length of the surgery (which may be less with an experienced surgeon), size of the mass (if a myoma/septum or polyp is present), the size of the endometrial cavity (if endometrial ablation or resection is performed), and the length of the procedure. It is also believed that preoperative treatment with one of the various hormonal agents may improve surgery, in some cases because of the reduction in endometrial or myoma vascularity (see Chapter 7).

Molnar and coworkers retrospectively evaluated 300 patients

who underwent endometrial resection to determine the most significant factors predisposing to increased levels of intravasation, in an attempt to devise a scoring system to predict patients at risk from fluid overload (18). They found the following factors significantly increased the amount of fluid intravasation in patients undergoing endometrial ablation, via resection: nulliparity; type of preoperative endometrial preparation; increased uterine size; increased cavity length; concurrent hysteroscopic myomectomy; and duration of surgery. In contrast to other reports, tubal patency and the use of an intracervical injection of a vasoconstricting substance had no significant effect on fluid balance.

After evaluation of these multiple factors, their final conclusion was ". . . as it is impossible to predict all cases of fluid overload, it is still imperative that fluid balance is monitored closely in all patients undergoing hysteroscopic surgery" (18).

Garry and colleagues described two different mechanisms by which they believe fluid absorption may occur (19). Based on studies during Nd–YAG laser ablations, they concluded that when superficial layers of the endometrium are coagulated, fluid absorption is proportional to intrauterine pressure, whereas deep destruction or tissue injury allows larger blood vessels and/or sinus tracts to open, allowing fluid absorption regardless of the level of intrauterine pressure.

Several studies have evaluated fluid loss with controlled pressure systems. In a prospective randomized study, Hasham and coworkers found no fluid absorption when using the Hamou hysteromat (Karl Storz, Endoscopy) versus 1255 cc per case of absorption in the non-pressure controlled group (20). (This device is not yet approved for sale in the United States.)

In another interesting study, Vulgaropulos and colleagues evaluated intrauterine pressures and flow rates in an in vitro system (21). They found these parameters affected by: (1) height of the media or pump setting; (2) hysteroscope manufacturer; (3) amount of cervical dilation; and (4) whether the outflow valve was opened or closed. In an in vivo evaluation of fifteen patients, they evaluated fluid absorption of 1.5% glycine with 2% ethanol by several methods, including hematocrit, plasma sodium and osmolarity, and blood ethanol levels.

Interestingly, they found no significant change in any of these parameters and contrary to other published reports, intrauterine pressure above 200 mmHg did not result in significant fluid absorption.

Although previous reports of ethanol use in irrigating fluids have been published in the anesthesiology literature, this was the first application to hysteroscopic surgery (22).

COMPLICATIONS OF LOW VISCOSITY MEDIA

The most significant complication of low viscosity fluids is their ability to cause fluid overload and, in the case of hypotonic fluids, to additionally cause dilution hyponatremia. Decades ago, urologists described a syndrome of dilution hyponatremia later called the postTUR (transurethral resection) syndrome, because of its association with prostatic resection. This syndrome includes initial bradycardia and hypertension followed by nausea, vomiting, hypertension, seizures, pulmonary edema, and cardiac decompensation. Coma and death have now been reported in both the urologic and gynecologic literature (6).

As previously described, the solutions most commonly used for resectoscopy are hypotonic. An understanding of plasma osmolarity and the impact of sodium levels are critically important. The equation

$$2 \times Na + glucose / 18 + Bun /28$$

is a close approximation of serum osmolarity. As can be seen from the equation, in the normal physiologic state, a significant percentage of the serum osmolarity is accounted for by sodium. During resectoscopic surgery using glycine as a medium, glycine enters the vascular system. It does have an osmolarity (200 mosm/L), although lower than serum. Because of glycine's short half-life, it is rapidly metabolized, leaving only free water in its place. This helps to explain the clinical scenario of a patient who is stable during the initial postop period, becoming symptomatic several hours after the completion of surgery. As the glycine (which has an osmotic effect) is removed from the circulation, the overall osmolarity is decreased (Figure 5-8). This allows an understanding of why the ideal medium would be isotonic. Isotonicity does not obviate the problem of fluid overload but does decrease the potential of fluid shifts between

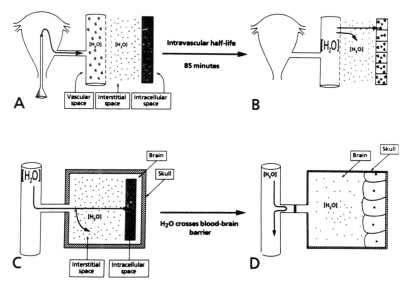

FIGURE 5-8

Cerebral edema following absorption of glycine irrigating solution. (A) Intravascular osmolarity is initially maintained by glycine molecules [G] contained in the intravascular space. (B) When glycine moves from the intravascular space into the cell, intravascular osmolarity falls. The concentration of water (H_2O) is greater in the intravascular space than in the interstitial space. As a result, water moves from the vascular space into the interstitial and intracellular space (arrows). (C) Because of the intravascular hypo-osmolar state, water moves across the blood-brain barrier into the interstitial and intracellular space. (D) Cerebral edema develops with compression of the brain against the skull. Water will continue to move into the brain until the hydrostatic pressure of the brain offsets the osmotic force. Reproduced with permission from Witz CA, Silverberg KM, Burns WN, Schenken RS, Olive DL. Complicaptions associated with the absorption of hysterscopic fluid media. Fertil Steril 1993;60:745.

compartments. This becomes important because of the potential for cerebral edema with hypotonic fluids. The blood–brain barrier allows free movement of water. In situations of plasma hypo-osmolarity and normal brain tissue osmolarity, the flow of water would be into the tissue of higher osmolarity to effect an equilibrium. Unlike other tissues, the brain is almost completely enclosed within the skull. Cerebral edema will cause the brain to press on the cranium, possibly decreasing cerebral blood flow, increasing intracranial pressure, leading to potential tissue hypoxia. Baggish and coworkers reported on two cases of hyponatremia using 3% sorbitol and 1.5% glycine (6). In one case, the patient's serum sodium was 121 mmol/L, in the second case, 102 mmol/L. In both cases, coma, respiratory arrest, and death ensued. Postmortem examination revealed cerebral herniation in both cases.

Mannitol has been suggested as a safer fluid because of its higher osmolarity (6). Although mannitol has no electrolytes and, thus, may also produce hyponatremia, it has a higher endogenous osmotic effect (274 mosm/L). Evaluation of its metabolism shows it is excreted, essentially unconverted, through the kidneys. This produces an osmotic diuresis, and theoretically, the free water, which would have been left intravascularly, is pulled with the mannitol, allowing a steady-state osmolality and decreasing the potential risks of cerebral edema.

Arieff and colleagues have suggested that premenopausal women may be at a higher risk from hyponatremia (23). He believes the sodium-potassium pump in the brain is altered by the presence or absence of estrogen and cites this as an explanation for the increased morbidity and mortality of hyponatremia in premenopausal women than in men or postmenopausal women. Progesterone has also been suggested as an additional modifier of this system (24). This might have implications on what pretreatment regimen a patient is placed on.

The relative role of hypo-osmolarity, hyponatremia, or their combination in the level of morbidity remains to be elucidated. Sodium is well known to have many physiologic effects, besides being a major constituent of the osmotic pressure. In an animal model, serum osmolarity was held at normal levels while intravascular sodium was markedly decreased (9). The investigators noted symptoms similar to the TUR syndrome in humans, including lethargy, convulsions, and coma.

Treatment of Hyponatremia

Early detection and initiation of treatment are important aspects in treating hyponatremia and fluid overload. Table 5-4 lists the steps in managing cases of acute hyponatremia. If hyponatremia is suspected, surgery should be immediately stopped. A loop diuretic, such as furosemide (20 mg IV—if there is no renal impairment), should be administered. This initiates a rapid diuresis, which aids in decreasing intravascular free water. Although hyponatremia was historically treated by fluid restriction and observation, this is inappropriate for acute surgically-induced hyponatremia, which the clinician encounters during or following hysteroscopy. Concomitant with diuretic administration, electrolytes should be sent immediately. Depending on the results, electrolytes should be repeated every several hours until sodium and potassium are normalized. With increasing degrees of volume overload and/or hyponatremia, central monitoring may become important in accessing the complex hemodynamics that may occur. Normal saline may be used for sodium repletion, as hypertonic saline may cause an overshoot of

---

TABLE 5-4

Steps in the Treatment of Hyponatremia

Stop procedure
Diuretic to reduce hypervolemia
Send electrolytes STAT
Central venous monitoring
Normal saline for repletion
Close monitoring of input/output
Steady increases in serum sodium

---

sodium levels with subsequent hypernatremia. Close evaluation of systemic parameters, including urine output, blood pressure, cardiac status, and restriction of input, are necessary. Serial electrolytes should demonstrate a steady increase and ultimate stabilization of sodium. It is important to note that there is a mortality rate for acute hyponatremia even at levels previously thought to be acceptable. In the report by Baggish and colleagues on media toxicity, one of the deaths occurred in a patient with serum sodium of 121 mmol/L (6).

Treatment should take into account whether the situation is acute (as most surgical cases will be) or chronic (>48 hours). In acute cases, many authors have suggested increases of 1-2 meq/L per hour for the first 6 hours is adequate and may have a significant impact on the level of cerebral edema (25–27). In cases where hyponatremia is immediately recognized, it is likely that even quicker repletion of sodium is possible.

Cases of chronic hyponatremia appear to have less morbidity and mortality at similar levels. However, it is now well recognized that correcting chronic hyponatremia too rapidly may lead to a clinical entity referred to as central pontine myelinolysis (CPM). A conceptualization of the pathogenesis is presented in Figure 5-9. As with acute hyponatremia, ineffective repletion of sodium may lead to persistent or worsening symptoms. Chronic hyponatremia, like acute hyponatremia, should be slowly but effectively treated. An increase of 1 meq/L every 2 hours helps to protect against development of CPM. In addition, use of hypertonic saline may predispose the patient to CPM by too quickly correcting serum sodium.

Use of mannitol as a diuretic for acute or chronic hyponatremia remains unclear, since osmotic diuresis will occur—but at the expense of further exacerbating fluid overload.

COMPLICATIONS OF HIGH VISCOSITY MEDIA

Because of Hyskon's high molecular weight and extended half-life, fluid problems and treatments associated with intravasation are much

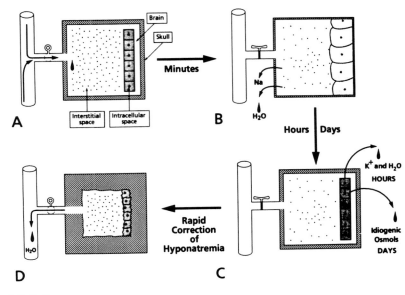

FIGURE 5-9

Pathogenesis of central pontine myelinolysis. (A) As a result of intravascular hypo-osmolarity, water moves into the brain. The brain swells and is compressed against the skull. (B) Within minutes, sodium and water are extruded from the extracellular space into the cerebrospinal fluid and, ultimately, into the vasculature. (C) To decrease swelling, the brain cells release potassium and "idiogenic osmols." The brain now has decreased the number of osmotically active particles. This response takes up to several days. (D) A rapid increase in plasma osmolarity (as with rapid correction of hyponatremia) leads to movement of water out of the brain and into the vascular space, causing desiccation of the brain. Reproduced with permission from Witz CA, Silverberg KM, Burns WN, Schenken RS, Olive DL. Complications associated with the absorption of hysteroscopic fluid media. Fertil Steril 1993;60:745.

different from low viscosity fluids. In addition, Hyskon is associated with a number of unique problems. Hyskon is a relatively heterogeneous fluid in which the average molecular weight is 70 kd but may contain units with both smaller or larger molecular weights. This has metabolic importance, since particles <50 kd are renally excreted, whereas larger compounds are metabolized via the reticuloendo-

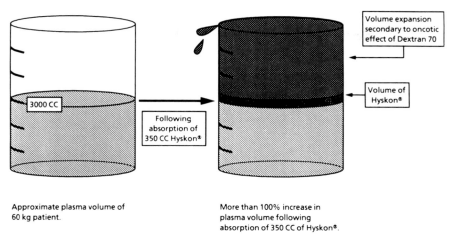

Approximate plasma volume of 60 kg patient.

More than 100% increase in plasma volume following absorption of 350 CC of Hyskon®.

FIGURE 5-10

Plasma volume expansion resulting from the absorption of 350 mL of Hyskon. The volume is increased by 350 mL of Hyskon plus 3,000 mL of fluid that is drawn osmotically into the intravascular space. Note that plasma volume is increased by >100%. Reproduced with permission from Witz CA, Silverberg KM, Burns WN, Schenken RS, Olive DL. Complications associated with the absorption of hysteroscopic fluid media. Fertil Steril 1993;60:745.

thelial system. Because of the limited acute metabolism and ability to function as an osmotic particle within the intravascular space, significant increases in intravascular volume may occur, even with limited intravasation. Figure 5-10 demonstrates the intravascular effect of absorbing 350 cc of Hyskon. This is the rationale for many authorities recommending that total loss not exceed 300 cc, and package labeling recommending less than 500 cc total loss.

In contrast to low viscosity fluids where intravasation leads to hypo-osmolar plasma, intravasation of Hyskon causes an increase in plasma oncotic pressure, which draws in fluid from the extravascular spaces. In both situations, significant volume overload may occur. The difference lies in the causal mechanism. Multiple reports have demonstrated the ability of Hyskon to induce pulmonary edema through the aforementioned mechanism (28). What is unclear is at what amount of intravasation do the risks of pulmonary edema become significant? It is likely that age, cardiopulmonary status, renal function, and other multiple factors predispose subsets of patients, while most healthy patients would likely tolerate a greater degree of overload. Baggish and coworkers evaluated the relationship between the volume of Hyskon administered and Hyskon blood levels during hysteroscopy in an attempt to predict a threshold for toxicity (29). They found a poor correlation between amount of Hyskon used and blood levels at 30 minutes and found uptake increased in patients with the greatest myometrial and endometrial damage.

Some authors have suggested a direct effect of dextran on the pulmonary vasculature (30,31). They believe this toxic effect occurs at the level of the pulmonary capillaries, allowing fluid leakage and subsequent pulmonary edema. While there is evidence for such a cause/effect relationship for several other medications (dextran 40, ritodrine, opiates, and salicylates), scientific consensus on this effect for dextran 70 is unclear (32,33).

Treatment for excess intravascular Hyskon, which causes pulmonary edema, is debatable. Use of diuretics, ventilatory support, and central venous monitoring are important. Unfortunately, the high molecular weight of Hyskon does not allow renal diuresis of the dextran 70 particles. Supportive management until the reticulo-endothelial system clears the Hyskon is warranted. Some authors have advocated plasmapheresis for protracted cases with elevated plasma oncotic pressure, such as that produced by excess Hyskon, but little information is available (34). Such difficult cases are best handled in consultation with nephrologists and intensive-care specialists.

Hyskon has been associated with changes in the coagulation cascade (35). It has been suggested that such coagulation inhibition may contribute to postoperative bleeding or hemoptysis (36). While reports of disseminated intravascular coagulation secondary to hysteroscopic use of dextran are rare, reports of changes in clotting factors have been published (37). Baggish and colleagues found Hyskon decreased fibrinogen with no change in fibrin-split products (29). A much older report in the European literature demonstrated that Hyskon caused a reduction in platelet adhesiveness and aggregation (38).

Hyskon has also been associated with anaphylactic or allergic reactions (39). Even though Hyskon has little immunogenicity, there may be cross-reactivity to the antigen in other dextran-containing substances, such as turnips, beets, or, possibly, bacterial antigens. These idiosyncratic reactions may range from minor allergic manifestations, such as skin changes, to cardiac collapse (14,39). While often discussed, it is felt that the true incidence of this complication is small (40). Treatment is similar to that of an allergic reaction.

Because Hyskon is significantly hypertonic, the clinician must carefully monitor the amount of fluid used to decrease the possibility of intravascular absorption. Most authors have recommended total fluid to be used to be between 350 cc and 500 cc. However, as Figure 5-10 demonstrated, even a small amount of Hyskon loss leads to significant fluid shifts and volume expansion within the intravascular space. In addition, anaphylactic reactions are unrelated to amount of use, and there seems no effective way to predict who may react to these agents. Interestingly, several patients who exhibited allergic responses were later tested for allergy to dextran and found to be negative (39,40). Like low viscosity fluids, Hyskon may be successfully utilized in a number of clinical scenarios to effectively distend the uterus. Familiarity with the potential problems will allow the astute clinician to avert problems and manage them in an appropriate and timely fashion when they occur.

CLINICAL PEARLS

✖ No perfect medium exists; clinicians must be familiar with a number of media, their risks, and benefits.

✖ Carbon dioxide should only be instilled via a dedicated hysteroscopic insufflator.

✖ Normal saline and lactated Ringer's are not useful media when using unipolar current, such as with the resectoscope.

✖ Use of sterile water as a medium is inappropriate as it causes hemolysis if intravasation occurs.

✖ Glycine and sorbitol are commonly used distention

media when electrosurgery is employed—both are hypotonic and may induce hyponatremia if excess intravasation occurs.

✖ ALWAYS monitor input and output every 10–15 minutes throughout cases.

✖ NEVER assume that fluid on the floor makes up the deficit.

✖ ALWAYS check electrolytes if overload is suspected.

✖ Hyskon is very hypertonic, and intravasation of small amounts may cause significant intravascular expansion.

✖ Excess intrauterine pressure increases fluid intravasation risk without benefiting distention and visualization.

✖ It is currently difficult to monitor intrauterine pressure, and thus, the least pressure to distend the cavity and facilitate surgery should be used.

✖ Multiple factors may affect the risk of intravasation, including surgeon experience, uterine size, length of the procedure, and endometrial preparation.

✖ Chronic hyponatremia should be corrected slowly, but continuously, to decrease the risk of central pontine myelinolysis.

✖ The best method of treatment for hyponatremia is avoidance through close attention to fluid status. Early recognition and prompt treatment with a diuretic are critical.

REFERENCES

1. Rubin IC. Uterine endoscopy, endometroscopy with the aid of uterine insufflation. Am J Obstet Gynecol 1925;10:313.
2. Rubin IC. Uterotubal insufflation. St. Louis: CV Mosby, 1947.
3. Baggish MS, Daniel JF. Death caused by air embolism associated with neodymium:yttrium aluminum–garnet laser surgery and artificial sapphire tips. Am J Obstet Gynecol 1989;161:877–888.

4. Madsen PO, Madsen RE. Clinical and experimental evaluation of different irrigating fluids for transurethral surgery. Invest Urol 1965; 3:122–129.

5. Dequesne J. Hysteroscopic treatment of uterine bleeding with the Nd-YAG laser. Lasers in Medical Science 1987;2:73–76.

6. Baggish MS, Brill AI, Rosensweig B, Barbot JE, Indman P. Fatal acute glycine and sorbitol toxicity during operative hysteroscopy. J Gynecol Surg 1993;9:137–143.

7. Weiner J, Gregory L. Absorption of irrigating fluid during transcervical resection of endometrium. British Med J 1990;300:748–749.

8. Roesch RP, Stoelting RK, Lingeman JE, Kahnoski JR, Bacakes DJ, Gephardt SA. Ammonia toxicity resulting from glycine absorption during transurethral resection of the prostate. Anesthesiology 1983; 58:577–579.

9. Berstein GT, Loughlin KR, Gittes RF. The physiologic basis for the TURP syndrome. J Surg Res 1989;46:135–141.

10. Mizutani AR, Parker J, Katz J, Schmidt J. Visual disturbances, serum glycine levels, and transurethral resection of the prostate. J Urol 1990;144:697–699.

11. Duffy S, Sharp F, Reid P. Irrigation solutions and blood: the electrical events during electrosurgery. Gynecol Endocrinol 1992;1:11–14.

12. Edstrom K, Fernstrom I. The diagnostic possibilities of a modified hysteroscopic technique. Acta Obstet Gynecol Scand 1970;49:327–330.

13. Amin HK, Neuwirth RS. Operative hysteroscopy utilizing dextran as a distending medium. Clin Obstet Gynecol 1983;26:277–284.

14. Loffer FD. Complications from uterine distention during hysteroscopy. In: Corfman KS, Diamond MP, DeCherney A, eds. Complications in laparoscopy and hysteroscopy. Boston: Blackwell Scientific Publications, 1993:177–186.

15. Baumann R, Magos AC, Kayo JOS, Turnbull AC. Absorption of glycine irrigating fluid during transcervical resection of the endometrium. Br Med J 1990;300:304–305.

16. Magos AL, Baumann R, Turnbull AC. Safety of transcervical endometrial resection. Lancet 1990;355:44.

17. Lomano JM. Photocoagulation of the endometrium with the Nd-YAG laser for the treatment of menorrhagia. J Reprod Med 1986;31:148–150.

18. Molnar BG, Broadbent JAM, Magos AL. Fluid overload risk score for endometrial resection. Gynecol Endocrinol 1992;1:133–138.

19. Garry R, Mooney P, Hasham F, Kokri M. A uterine distention system to prevent fluid absorption during Nd-YAG laser endometrial ablation. Gynecol Endocrinol 1992;1:23–27.

20. Hasham F, Garry R, Kokri MS, Mooney P. Fluid absorption during laser ablation of the endometrium in the treatment of menorrhagia. Br J Anaesth 1992;68:151–154.

21. Vulgaropulos SP, Haley LC, Hulka JF. Intrauterine pressure and fluid absorption during continuous flow hysteroscopy. Am J Obstet Gynecol 1992;167:386–391.

22. Hahn RG. Ethanol monitoring of irrigating fluid absorption in transurethral prostatic surgery. Anesthesiology 1988;68:867–873.

23. Arieff AI. Hyponatremia, convulsions, respiratory arrest, and permanent brain damage after elective surgery in healthy women. N Engl J Med 1986;314:1529–1535.

24. Berl T. Treating hyponatremia: what is the controversy about? Ann Intern Med 1990;113:417–419.

25. Witz CA, Silverberg KM, Burns WN, Schenken RS, Olive DL. Complications associated with the absorption of hysteroscopic fluid media. Fertil Steril 1993;60:745–756.

26. Sterns RH. The management of symptomatic hyponatremia. Semin Nephrol 1990;10:503–514.

27. Sterns RH. The treatment of hyponatremia: first, do no harm. Am J Med 1990;88:557–560.

28. Schinagl EF. Hyskon (32% dextran 70) hysteroscopic surgery and pulmonary edema. Anesth Anal 1990;70:223–224.

29. Baggish MS, Davaulur C, Rodriguez F, Comporesi E. Vascular uptake of Hyskon (dextran 70) during operative and diagnostic hysteroscopy. J Gynecol Surg 1992;8:211–217.

30. Zbella EA, Moise J, Carson SA. Noncardiogenic pulmonary edema secondary to intrauterine instillation of 32% dextran 70. Fertil Steril 1985;43:479–480.

31. Leake J, Murphy AA, Zacur H. Noncardiogenic pulmonary edema: a complication of operative hysteroscopy. Fertil Steril 1987;48:497–499.

32. Kaplan AI, Sabin S. Dextran 40: another cause of drug-induced noncardiogenic pulmonary edema. Chest 1975;68:376–377.

33. Benedetti TJ. Maternal complications of parenteral B-sympathomimetic therapy for premature labor. Am J Obstet Gynecol 1983;145:1–6.

34. Moran M, Kapsner C. Acute renal failure associated with elevated plasma oncotic pressure. N Engl J Med 1987;317:150–153.
35. Ljungstrom KG. Safety of 32% dextran for hysteroscopy. Am J Obstet Gynecol 1990;163:2029–2030.
36. Siegler AM, Valle RF, Lindemann HJ, Mencaglia L. In: Therapeutic hysteroscopy indications and techniques. St. Louis: CV Mosby, 1990:51.
37. Jedekin R, Kessler I, Olsfanger D. Disseminated intravascular coagulopathy and adult respiratory distress syndrome: life-threatening complications of hysteroscopy. Am J Obstet Gynecol 1990;162:44–45.
38. Cronberg S, Robertson B, Nilsson IM, Nilehn JE. Suppressive effect of dextran on platelet adhesiveness. Thrombos Diasthes Haemorrh 1966;16:384–392.
39. Trimbos-Kemper TCM, Veering BT. Anaphylactic shock from intracavitary 32% dextran 70 during hysteroscopy. Fertil Steril 1989;51:1053–1054.
40. Ahmed N, Falcone T, Tulandi T, Houle G. Anaphylactic reaction because of intrauterine 32% dextran 70 instillation. Fertil Steril 1991;55:1014–1016.

6

Preoperative Evaluation for Resectoscopic Surgery

Randall Barnes

I t is a well accepted axiom that a successful outcome in surgery depends on appropriate preoperative evaluation to establish the correct diagnosis and to determine the appropriate surgical therapy. A successful surgical outcome also depends upon proper preoperative patient preparation. This chapter will consider the preoperative evaluation of patients presenting for resectoscopic surgery, appropriate preoperative preparation with regard to prophylactic antibiotics, preparation of the cervix for dilation, and anesthesia.

PREOPERATIVE EVALUATION

Common uses of the gynecologic resectoscope include incision of a uterine septum, lysis of intrauterine adhesions, removal of intrauterine growths, and endometrial ablation. Patients with a uterine septum usually present with a history of recurrent spontaneous abortion. Evaluation of the uterine cavity by hysterosalpingogram or hysteroscopy is essential in the workup of recurrent spontaneous abortion. If a septum is present, transvaginal ultrasound can often distinguish between a septate and bicornuate uterus. In doubtful cases, a laparoscopy should be done either before or at the time of a septal lysis to confirm a septate uterus. Postoperatively, a hysteroscopy or hysterosalpingogram is useful to determine whether or not the uterine cavity is normal. Occasionally, the septal lysis is incomplete and a second surgery is necessary.

Patients requiring therapy of Asherman's syndrome usually result from an investigation of recurrent pregnancy wastage or infertility. In the United States, the great majority of patients acquire Asherman's syndrome as a result of a curettage of a pregnant or recently pregnant uterus. A less common cause is uterine surgery, such as myomectomy. About half of patients with Asherman's syndrome present with a history of infertility and about half with a history of recurrent pregnancy loss (1). The menstrual history is not particularly useful in establishing the diagnosis, as patients with extensive adhesions can present with eumenorrhea, hypomenorrhea, or amenorrhea. Hysterosalpingogram is vital to determine the extent of adhesions preoperatively and, postoperatively, to confirm the success of the procedure.

Evaluation of Abnormal Uterine Bleeding

Abnormal uterine bleeding is an extremely common problem. In England, about 30 per 1000 female patients per year consult with their general practitioners for evaluation of abnormal uterine bleeding. About 20% of referrals from general practitioners to gynecologists are for abnormal uterine bleeding, and of those referred, about half undergo hysterectomy (2). Because of the high incidence of abnormal bleeding and likelihood of hysterectomy, proper evaluation and consideration of nonsurgical therapies are essential to the management of abnormal uterine bleeding.

The critical distinction to be made in the evaluation of abnormal uterine bleeding is whether it is associated with ovulation or anovulation. For the purposes of this chapter, abnormal uterine bleeding associated with anovulation will be referred to as *dysfunctional uterine bleeding* (DUB). *Menorrhagia* is defined as heavy menses in ovulatory women, while *metrorrhagia* is irregular bleeding during an ovulatory cycle (Table 6-1). The distinction between ovulatory and anovulatory bleeding is critical because causes and therapies are distinct.

TABLE 6-1

Causes of Abnormal Uterine Bleeding

Menometrorrhagia

    Anatomic

        Leiomyomata

        Endometrial polyp

        Adenomyosis

    IUD

    Bleeding disorders

        von Willebrand's disease

        Platelet disorders

    Hypothyroidism

    Essential menorrhagia

Dysfunctional Uterine Bleeding

    Physiologic

        Perimenarcheal and perimenopausal anovulation

    Hypothalamic dysfunction

        Stress

        Exercise

        Weight loss

    Androgen excess

        Polycystic ovary syndrome

        Late onset 21-hydroxylase deficiency

    Hypothyroidism

    Consequences of chronic anovulation

        Endometrial hyperplasia

        Endometrial cancer

Menometrorrhagia

The diagnosis of menorrhagia, or heavy menstrual bleeding, is usually made by the patient. Menstrual bleeding lasting longer than seven days or associated with clotting is common in menorrhagia.

The average menstrual blood loss is about 40 mL per cycle; any loss greater than 80 mL is associated with an increase risk of anemia and is considered menorrhagia (3,4). Because accurate measurement of menstrual blood loss is inconvenient and cumbersome, the diagnosis of menorrhagia is subjective, and often, the only objective indicator available to the physician is an abnormally low hemoglobin.

Metrorrhagia may be physiologic when it presents as midcycle spotting, which is probably the result of falling estradiol levels during the time of the luteinizing hormone surge. Any other metrorrhagia is abnormal and deserves investigation.

Menometrorrhagia is often difficult to distinguish from dysfunctional uterine bleeding. Ovulation should be confirmed in all cases by a serum progesterone greater than 3 ng/mL or finding secretory endometrium on biopsy. Basal body temperature charting is useful to time the above tests (Table 6-2).

Causes of Menometrorrhagia

Uterine leiomyomata, particularly those that distort the uterine cavity, endometrial polyps, and adenomyosis are common anatomic abnormalities causing menometrorrhagia. In women undergoing hysteroscopy for menorrhagia, 10 to 15% had submucosal fibroids and 15 to 30% had endometrial polyps (5). Adenomyosis was found in hysteroscopic biopsy specimens in 37% of 90 menorrhagic women. If the uterine cavity was normal, 66% had significant adenomyosis (5). Adenomyosis was found in 46% of 43 women with an enlarged uterus without evidence of leiomyomata on ultrasound who had hysterectomy for recurrent menorrhagia (6).

All IUDs, with the exception of those containing progestins, increase the prevalence of menorrhagia. Depending on the type used, menorrhagia occurs in 25 to 50% of IUD users after one year (4). Hypothyroidism causes a range of menstrual abnormalities from amenorrhea to menometrorrhagia (7). Early hypothyroidism has been found in 22% of women with menorrhagia (8). Overt hypothyroidism was found in 2% of women with menorrhagia evaluated for endometrial ablation (5).

Although it is uncommon for bleeding disorders to present to

TABLE 6-2

Evaluation of Abnormal Uterine Bleeding

All Patients

Pregnancy test

CBC

TSH

Platelet count, PT, PTT, and bleeding time (if coagulation disorder suspected)

Ovulatory versus Anovulatory

Endometrial biopsy

Serum progesterone

Basal body temperature

Ovulatory Bleeding (Menometrorrhagia)

Transvaginal ultrasound, hysterosalpingogram, or hysteroscopy

Endometrial biopsy (if over 40 years old)

Anovulatory Bleeding (Dysfunctional Uterine Bleeding)

Prolactin, FSH

If androgen excess present: testosterone, free testosterone, 8 AM 17-hydroxyprogesterone

If anovulatory for more than one year: endometrial biopsy

If unresponsive to medical therapy: rule out anatomic defect

the gynecologist with abnormal uterine bleeding, the possibility should always be considered. Von Willebrand's disease has been found in patients considered for endometrial ablation (5). In particular, bleeding disorders should be considered in adolescents admitted to the hospital with acute menorrhagia. A primary coagulation disorder has been reported in almost 20% of such patients with 50% of patients hospitalized with excessive bleeding at menarche having clotting disorders. Von Willebrand's disease and platelet abnormalities, such as idiopathic thrombocytopenia, were the most commonly found disorders (9).

Essential menorrhagia is the final cause of menorrhagia. It has been reported to occur in about 10% of western European women (4). Since it is a diagnosis of exclusion, it may be difficult to distinguish from adenomyosis.

Evaluation of Menometrorrhagia

The patient presenting with menometrorrhagia should be evaluated for the presence of an anatomic abnormality (Table 6-2). Oftentimes, this is easily accomplished by palpating a fibroid uterus on physical examination. However, symptomatic submucosal fibroids can be present in a normal size uterus (Figure 6-1). Therefore, all patients should undergo transvaginal ultrasound, hysterosalpingogram or office hysteroscopy. A normal transvaginal ultrasound or hysterosalpingogram reliably rules out an intrauterine lesion (10,11). However, if a lesion is present, hysteroscopy is more reliable for distinguishing a polyp from a fibroid and determining the exact location and extent of the mass. Recently, intrauterine instillation of distention media hysterosalpingosonography (HSSG) has been suggested as a method to enhance sonographic examination of the uterine cavity. In one study comparing HSSG to hysteroscopy and hysterosalpingography (HSG), results demonstrated HSSG to be more sensitive but less specific than hysteroscopy or HSG (12).

The preoperative diagnosis of adenomyosis is more difficult to make. The physical finding of a diffusely enlarged, tender uterus is not always present. Recently, transvaginal ultrasound has been found to be about 80% sensitive in detecting adenomyosis with a 26% false-positive rate (6). The most reliable preoperative method for detecting adenomyosis is magnetic resonance imaging (13). However, this procedure is expensive and cannot currently be

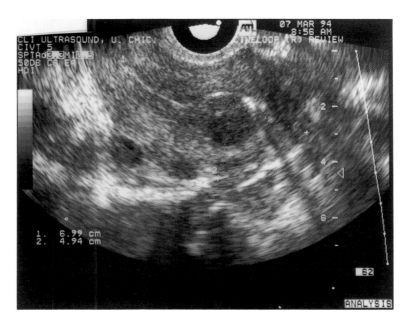

FIGURE 6-1

Transvaginal ultrasound demonstrates a 3-cm intracavity fibroid in a patient with normal uterine size who presented with menometrorrhagia.

recommended as part of the evaluation for every patient with menorrhagia.

Thyroid-stimulating hormone (TSH) should be measured in all patients with menorrhagia. If there is suspicion of a clotting disorder, a prothrombin time, partial thromboplastin time, platelet count, and clotting time should be done. Endometrial biopsy should be considered, particularly in women over 40, to rule out endometrial hyperplasia or cancer.

Medical Therapy of Menometrorrhagia

Resectoscopic removal of a submucosal fibroid or polyp in patients with menometrorrhagia who have not completed childbearing or otherwise wish to keep their uterus has rapidly become standard practice. In patients with menorrhagia, no anatomic abnormality, and no desire for fertility, ablation of the endometrium is a possible therapy. However, it must be emphasized that these patients require proper evaluation as outlined above. If hypothyroidism is present, patients respond very quickly to thyroid hormone replacement therapy with a rapid decline in menstrual blood loss (7,14). If deep adenomyosis is felt to be present, most authors believe that a hysterectomy, and not ablation, is a more appropriate therapy. Adenomyosis is a frequent finding in hysterectomy specimens from patients failing ablation (15,16).

Medical therapy is often effective for treating essential menorrhagia and should be attempted before an ablation. The oral contraceptive pill decreases menstrual blood loss by 50% (17). The progesterone-containing IUD is extremely effective in reducing menstrual blood loss. Although not available in the United States, a norgestrel–releasing IUD reduced menstrual blood loss by 96% after 12 months in patients with essential menorrhagia (18). The progesterone IUD, which is available in the United States, reduces blood loss by 65% after one year (19). Danazol 200 mg daily for 3 months has been reported to reduce menstrual blood loss by 80% (20).

Antiprostaglandins reduce menstrual blood loss by 20 to 50% (4,18,21,22). Systemic antifibrinolytic agents like tranexamic acid and epsilon aminocaproic acid have been used in Europe and reduce menstrual blood loss by 50% (4,17). However, side effects of these agents, such as nausea, diarrhea, and dizziness, limit their usefulness. In addition, at least three cases of intracranial arterial thrombosis have been described in women using antithrombolytics for menorrhagia (4). In the author's view, they should not be considered as an alternative to endometrial ablation.

Recently, gonadotropin-releasing hormone (GnRH) agonists have been investigated in patients with essential menorrhagia or adenomyosis. There have been two reports of pregnancy following agonist therapy of severe adenomyosis (23,24). A GnRH agonist together with hormone replacement therapy has also been reported to effectively treat essential menorrhagia (25). Because of their expense, GnRH agonists should be reserved for use in women with essential menorrhagia or adenomyosis who are unresponsive to any other medical therapy and who wish to preserve childbearing.

Dysfunctional Uterine Bleeding

In the author's experience, any cause of anovulation with normal estrogen levels can present as DUB (Table 6-1). Anovulatory cycles are considered physiologic in the first year after menarche and in the perimenopause and do not require extensive hormonal evaluation (26). However, the cause of anovulatory cycles at other times in a woman's reproductive life should be investigated (Table 6-2). Prolactin and TSH should be measured in all patients with anovulation, whether they present with amenorrhea, oligomenorrhea, or DUB to rule out hyperprolactinemia and hypothyroidism. FSH should also be measured, as dysfunctional bleeding may occur during the transition to premature ovarian failure, just as it does at the time of physiologic menopause.

Dysfunctional uterine bleeding is a common symptom of androgen excess. In women with dysfunctional bleeding and evidence of hirsutism or acne, the diagnosis of polycystic ovary syndrome can be made by finding elevated total or free testosterone. Late-onset 21-hydroxylase deficiency is an uncommon cause of androgen excess, occurring in less than 5% of hyperandrogenic women. It can be reliably ruled out by finding an 8 AM 17-hydroxyprogesterone of less than 2 ng/ml (27,28).

If there is no evidence of hyperprolactinemia, hypothyroidism, premature ovarian failure, or androgen excess, patients with DUB fit into the category of hypothalamic dysfunction. They may be anovulatory due to stress, weight loss, exercise, or the cause may be idiopathic. These patients can be reassured that, as long as they continue to withdraw to a progestin challenge, there is no serious cause for their anovulation.

The long-term consequence of chronic anovulation is endometrial hyperplasia and carcinoma. An endometrial biopsy should be considered in all patients with anovulatory bleeding, particularly those over 40 years old. Some authors recommend that an endometrial biopsy be done in a patient of any age with a history of anovulatory bleeding of more than one year duration because there have been reports of endometrial cancer in patients as young as 15 years of age (26,29).

Treatment of Dysfunctional Uterine Bleeding

When DUB is due to hyperprolactinemia, a dopamine agonist, such as bromocriptine, is effective in restoring ovulatory function. Some hyperprolactinemic patients may be treated with periodic progestin withdrawal. Patients with DUB and hypothyroidism respond quickly to thyroid hormone replacement therapy, as noted above.

In other patients with hypothalamic dysfunction and dysfunctional uterine bleeding, periodic progestin administration is effective in restoring a normal bleeding pattern (Table 6-3). A progestin, such as medroxyprogesterone acetate, is given by mouth 5 mg daily for the first 13 days of each month. There is evidence that at least 13

TABLE 6-3

Medical Therapy of Abnormal Uterine Bleeding

Ovulatory Bleeding (Essential Menorrhagia)	
	Birth control pill
	Antiprostaglandins
	Antithrombolytics
	Danazol
	Progesterone IUD
Dysfunctional Uterine Bleeding	
	Acute episode
	Birth control pill
	IV conjugated equine estrogen
	Chronic control
	Monthly progestin
	Birth control pill

days of progestin therapy is necessary to eliminate the risk of endometrial hyperplasia (30). The birth control pill is also effective in patients with DUB. It is particularly useful in patients with polycystic ovary syndrome as it helps control symptoms of androgen excess.

Occasionally, patients with DUB present with acute episodes of extremely heavy bleeding that require immediate therapy. In these patients, progestins alone are not effective, and estrogen must also be given. An effective outpatient therapy is to give any low-dose oral contraceptive pill, one pill four times daily for 7 days. Patients usually stop bleeding within 12 to 24 hours, but therapy should be continued for the full 7 days. Upon completion of therapy, the patient will have a self-limited episode of bleeding, which may be heavy. Five days after discontinuing the four times a day dosage, the birth control pill can be restarted, one tablet daily as for contraception (31). In patients with significant anemia, the withdrawal bleed may be postponed by continuing the oral contraceptive until the hemoglobin is adequate to allow a withdrawal bleed. In women requiring inpatient observation and therapy, intravenous Premarin has been shown to be effective in the treatment of DUB; 25 mg is given every 3 to 4 hours for up to three doses (32). After treating the acute episode of bleeding, it is important to put patients on chronic intermittent progestin therapy or the birth control pill to prevent further episodes.

Endometrial ablation may not be the ideal therapy in patients with DUB, because chronic anovulation and unopposed ovarian estrogen production will continue despite ablation. Since the endometrium is not completely destroyed in all endometrial ablations, there is a continued need of progestin therapy to prevent endometrial carcinoma in the residual islands. A case of endometrial carcinoma has been reported in a patient five years after an endometrial ablation for DUB (33). Hysterectomy may be a more appropriate surgical choice for patients who cannot tolerate or do not respond to medical therapy for DUB and who have a normal endometrial cavity.

PREOPERATIVE CONSIDERATIONS IN RESECTOSCOPIC SURGERY

Preoperative considerations in patients undergoing resectoscopic surgery include the use of agents to cause endometrial atrophy, laminaria to aid cervical dilation, prophylactic antibiotics, and consideration of appropriate anesthesia during surgery. The question of preoperative endometrial preparation will be considered in Chapter 7.

A review of ten reports of hysteroscopic surgery for removal of intrauterine growths or for endometrial ablation published from 1990 to 1993 revealed a number of preoperative strategies (15,16, 34–41). Prophylactic antibiotics were used in four series, and the remaining six made no comment. The most commonly used prophylactic antibiotic was doxycycline. There was only one report of a post-surgical endometritis, and this occurred in a subject receiving prophylactic antibiotic (37). It is our practice to use prophylactic antibiotics in cases that are prolonged or require multiple transcervical insertions of the resectoscope.

Some authors recommend the insertion of laminaria the day before surgery because use of the resectoscope requires dilation of the cervix up to a 31 Hegar dilator (34,40). However, as with prophylactic antibiotics, there is no clear suggestion that laminaria use results in any consistent advantage or decreased likelihood of failure of the resectoscopic procedure. In patients with cervical stenosis or who are nulliparous, there may be a conceptual advantage to preoperative laminaria use.

The great majority of patients in these series received general anesthetic. However, regional anesthesia such as an epidural block, was used with equal success (16,36,39,40). One paper reported the use of intravenous sedation and paracervical block in 40 patients undergoing endometrial ablation (36). Only two of the 40 required additional anesthesia. Thus, conduction anesthesia as well as intravenous analgesia and pericervical block are effective for pain control for patients undergoing resectoscopic surgery.

CLINICAL PEARLS

✖ Menstrual history is a poor predictor of extent of intrauterine adhesions.

✖ Patients presenting for septal lysis with a history of miscarriage should be worked up for other causes prior to surgery.

✖ Uterine fibroids, endometrial polyps, and adenomyosis are common anatomic abnormalities causing menometrorrhagia.

✖ Preoperative diagnosis of adenomyosis is difficult.

✖ Evaluation of the uterine cavity, TSH, and possibly coagulation studies and endometrial biopsy are the core workup in patients with menorrhagia.

✖ Medical therapy is very effective in many patients with menorrhagia.

✖ In anovulatory patients, prolactin, TSH, and FSH should be evaluated. In patients with signs of hyperandrogenism, androgens should be evaluated.

✖ In anovulatory patients, endometrial biopsy should also be considered to rule out hyperplasia.

✖ In patients with acute heavy bleeds, estrogen must be given. Progestins are ineffective.

✖ It is unclear if prophylactic antibiotics are effective in decreasing infectious morbidity for hysteroscopy.

✖ Preoperative laminaria use has not yet been shown to be effective prior to hysteroscopy.

✖ General, regional, and paracervical blocks have all been effectively utilized as anesthetic regimens.

REFERENCES

1. Valle RF, Sciarra JJ. Intrauterine adhesions: hysteroscopic diagnosis, classification, treatment, and reproductive outcome. Am J Obstet Gynecol 1988;158:1459–1470.

2. Coulter A, Bradlow J, Agass M, Martin-Bates C, Tulloch A. Outcomes of referrals to gynaecology outpatient clinics for menstrual problems: an audit of general practice records. Br J Obstet Gynaecol 1991;98:789–796.

3. Hallberg L, Hogdahl AM, Nilson L, Rybo G. Menstrual blood loss—a population study. Acta Obstet Gynecol Scand 1966;45:320–351.

4. Eijkeren Van MA, Christiaens GCML, Sixma JJ, Haspels AA. Menorrhagia: a review. Obstet Gynecol Surv 1989;44:421–429.

5. McCausland AM. Hysteroscopic myometrial biopsy: its use in diagnosing adenomyosis and its clinical application. Am J Obstet Gynecol 1992;166:1619–1628.

6. Fedele L, Bianchi ST, Dorta M, Arcaini L, Zanotti F, Carinelli S. Transvaginal ultrasonography in the diagnosis of diffuse adenomyosis. Fertil Steril 1992;58:94–97.

7. Scott JC Jr, Mussey EL. Menstrual patterns in myxedema. Am J Obstet Gynecol 1964;90:161–165.

8. Wilansky DL, Greisman B. Early hypothyroidism in patients with menorrhagia. Am J Obstet Gynecol 1989;160:673–677.

9. Classens AE, Cowell CA. Acute adolescent menorrhagia. Am J Obstet Gynecol 1981;139:277–279.

10. Fayez JA, Mutie G, Schneider PJ. The diagnostic value of hysterosalpingography and hysteroscopy in infertility investigation. Am J Obstet Gynecol 1987;156:558–560.

11. Fedele L, Bianchi S, Dorta M, Brioschi D, Zanotti F, Vercellini P. Transvaginal ultrasonography versus hysteroscopy in the diagnosis of uterine submucous myomas. Obstet Gynecol 1991;77:745–748.

12. Bonilla-Musoles F, Simon C, Serra V, Sampaic M, Pellicar A. An assessment of hysterosalpingosonography (HSSG) as a diagnostic tool for uterine cavity defects and tubal patency. J Clin Ultrasound 1992;20:175–181.

13. Togashi K, Ozasa HI, Konishi I, et al. Enlarged uterus: differentiation

between adenomyosis and leiomyoma with MRI imaging. Radiology 1989;171:531–534.

14. Higham JM, Shaw RW. The effect of thyroxine replacement on menstrual blood loss in a hypothyroid patient. Br J Obstet Gynaecol 1992;99:695–696.

15. Derman SG, Rehnstrom J, Neuwirth RS. The long-term effectiveness of hysteroscopic treatment of menorrhagia and leiomyomas. Obstet Gynecol 1991;77:591–594.

16. Daniell JF, Kurtz BR, Ke RW. Hysteroscopic endometrial ablation using the rollerball electrode. Obstet Gynecol 1992;80:329–332.

17. Nilsson L, Rybo G. Treatment of menorrhagia. Am J Obstet Gynecol 1971;110:713–720.

18. Milson I, Anderson K, Andersch B, Rybo G. A comparison of flurbiprofen, tranexamic acid, and a levonorgestrel-releasing intrauterine contraceptive device in the treatment of idiopathic menorrhagia. Am J Obstet Gynecol 1991;164:879–883.

19. Bergqvist A, Sjukhuset A, Malmo RG. Treatment of menorrhagia with intrauterine release of progesterone. Br J Obstet Gynaecol 1983;90:255–258.

20. Chimbira TH, Anderson ABM, Naish C, Cope E, Turnbull AC. Reduction of menstrual blood loss by danazol in unexplained menorrhagia: lack of effect of placebo. Br J Obstet Gynaecol 1980;87:1152–1158.

21. Hall P, Maclachalan N, Thorn N, Nudd MWE, Taylor CG, Garrioch DB. Control of menorrhagia by the cyclo-oxygenase inhibitors naproxen sodium and mefenamic acid. Br J Obstet Gynaecol 1987;94:554–558.

22. van Eijkeren MA, Christiaens G, Geuze HJ, Haspels AA, Sixma JJ. Effects of mefenamic acid on menstrual hemostasis in essential menorrhagia. Am J Obstet Gynecol 1992;166:1419–1428.

23. Nelson JR, Corson SL. Long-term management of adenomyosis with a gonadotropin-releasing hormone agonist: a case report. Fertil Steril 1993;59:441–443.

24. Hirata JD, Moghissi KS, Ginsburg KA. Pregnancy after medical therapy of adenomyosis with a gonadotropin-releasing hormone agonist. Fertil Steril 1993;59:444–445.

25. Thomas EJ, Okuda KJ, Thomas NM. The combination of a depot

gonadotropin-releasing hormone agonist and cyclical hormone replacement therapy for dysfunctional uterine bleeding. Br J Obstet Gynaecol 1991;98:1155–1159.

26. Bayer SR, DeCherney AH. Clinical manifestations and treatment of dysfunctional uterine bleeding. JAMA 1993;269:1823–1828.

27. Azziz R, Zacur HA. 21-hydroxylase deficiency in female hyperandrogenism: screening and diagnosis. J Clin Endocrinol Metab 1989;69:577–584.

28. Ehrmann DA, Rosenfield RL, Barnes RB, Brigell DF, Sheikh Z. Detection of functional ovarian hyperandrogenism in women with androgen excess. N Engl J Med 1992;327:157–162.

29. Farhi DC, Nosanchuk J, Silverberg SG. Endometrial adenocarcinoma in women under 25 years of age. Obstet Gynecol 1986;68:741–745.

30. Mishell DR. Abnormal uterine bleeding. In: Herbst AR, Mishell DR, Stenchever MA, Droegemueller W, eds. Comprehensive gynecology. St. Louis: Mosby Year Book, 1992:1079–1099.

31. Dysfunctional uterine bleeding. In: Speroff L, Glass RH, Kase NG, eds. Clinical gynecologic endocrinology and infertility. Baltimore: Williams & Wilkins, 1989:265–282.

32. DeVore GR, Owens O, Kase N. Use of intravenous premarin in the treatment of dysfunctional uterine bleeding—a double-blind randomized control study. Obstet Gynecol 1982;59:285–291.

33. Copperman AB, DeCherney AH, Olive DL. A case of endometrial cancer following endometrial ablation for dysfunctional uterine bleeding. Obstet Gynecol 1993;82:640–642.

34. Townsend DE, Richart RM, Paskowitz RA, Woolfork RE. Instruments and methods. Obstet Gynecol 1990;76:310–313.

35. Loffer FD. Removal of large symptomatic intrauterine growths by the hysteroscopic resectoscope. Obstet Gynecol 1990;76:836–840.

36. Garry R, Erian J, Grochmal SA. A multi-centre collaborative study into the treatment of menorrhagia by Nd-YAG laser ablation of the endometrium. Br J Obstet Gynaecol 1991;98:357–362.

37. Corson SL, Brooks PG. Resectoscopic myomectomy. Fertil Steril 1991;55:1041–1044.

38. Pyper RJD, Haeri AD. A review of 80 endometrial resections for menorrhagia. Br J Obstet Gynaecol 1991;98:1049–1054.

39. VanDamme JP. One-stage endometrial ablation: results in 200 cases. Eur J Obstet Gynaecol Reprod Biol 1992;43:209–214.

40. Indman PD. Hysteroscopic treatment of menorrhagia associated with uterine leiomyomas. Obstet Gynecol 1993;81:716–720.

41. Dwyer N, Hutton J, Stirrat GM. Randomised controlled trial comparing endometrial resection with abdominal hysterectomy for the surgical treatment of menorrhagia. Br J Obstet Gynaecol 1993;100:237–243.

7

Uterine Preparation Prior to Surgery

Eric J. Bieber

T he concept of preparation of the uterus prior to surgery has received increasing attention as we strive to achieve higher success rates and facilitate our procedures. When DeCherney first reported on resectoscopic endometrial ablations, most of his patients were chronically sick with acute bleeding, and although there was no time for medical pretreatment, they achieved good results (1). As we have broadened the applications and indications of resectoscopic procedures, we see far less acute patients.

For the novice hysteroscopist, visualization is critical. There is nothing more frustrating to the beginning hysteroscopist than setting up the necessary equipment, only to insert the hysteroscope into a sea of blood and excess tissue that cannot be cleared. There are several preoperative and operative measures that will keep this experience to a minimum and potentially facilitate operative procedures.

The primary goals of pretreatment are to: (1) decrease the endometrial thickness; (2) decrease vascularity of the endometrium or myomata; (3) decrease blood loss at the time of surgery; (4) decrease operative time; (5) increase hemoglobin prior to surgery in anemic patients; (6) improve visualization and ease of surgery; and (7) possibly improve overall success and feasibility rates.

There are presently many different methods used in attempting to achieve these goals, ranging from appropriate timing during the cycle to medical or mechanical methods. Like many other applications in obstetrics and gynecology, none of the medical treatments discussed are approved as hysteroscopic endometrial pretreatments by the Food and Drug Administration. Once the FDA has approved a drug, physicians are not limited in their ability to use these agents for unlabeled applications. Such is the case with all medical agents discussed herein.

PRETREATMENT REGIMENS

Hysteroscopy during the Proliferative Phase

The simplest form of uterine preparation might be considered performance of a procedure during the early proliferative phase. Review of the endometrial height at various times during the menstrual cycle demonstrates the lowest or most basal endometrium following menses (Figure 7-1). An impressive increase in endometrial height occurs as a response to the endometrial mitogen estrogen. Diagnostic hysteroscopy is most easily performed after menses, prior to the excessive endometrial buildup, which occurs as early as the mid- to late proliferative phase. Performance of hysteroscopy during the luteal phase is more difficult, because disruption of endometrial tissue during hysteroscope insertion or manipulation often occurs. Excessive tissue may obscure intracavitary abnormalities and subtle lesions. In addition, luteal phase hysteroscopy carries the risk of disrupting a chemically undetectable pregnancy.

While we find the early proliferative phase an excellent time for diagnostic and simple operative procedures, on occasion, a surprising amount of tissue is present.

Progestational Agents

Progestins are commonly used in clinical practice to antagonize the effects of estrogen and initiate programmed endometrial changes, which allow a timed withdrawal bleed. These effects have been used

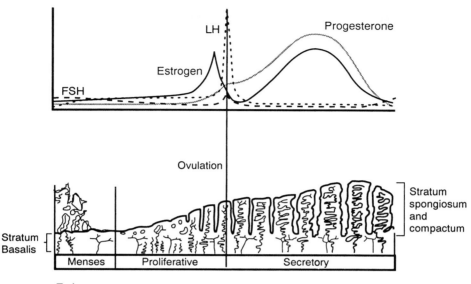

FIGURE 7-1

Demonstration of the change in endometrial height during the menstrual cycle.

to treat patients prior to hysteroscopic procedures. Progestins limit the growth of endometrium by multiple actions. When used over extended time periods, progestins induce pseudodecidual changes and eventual atrophy.

Multiple regimens have been used for this purpose, including depomedroxyprogesterone acetate (DMPA), oral medroxyprogesterone acetate, and norethindrone. In the depot formulation, DMPA is administered as a 150-mg intramuscular injection. Studies evaluating DMPA have found depo-injections to cause pharmacologic and contraceptive effects for at least 3 months (2). With the regimen of 150 mg every 3 months, approximately 50% of patients will become amenorrheic after one year and 60 to 70% amenorrheic after 2 years (3). This demonstrates the atrophy that ultimately takes place. Unfortunately, the effect is somewhat unpredictable, and approximately 10% of women have menorrhagia at 12 months (3).

Alternative regimens have used norethindrone 5 mg b.i.d. or

TABLE 7-1

Common Side Effects

GNRHA	DANAZOL	PROGESTINS
Hot flashes/sweats (80%)	Hot flashes/sweats (50–60%)	Menstrual abnormalities (25%)
Headaches (30%)	Androgen-like effects (30%)	Headache (15%)
		Abdominal discomfort (13%)
Vaginitis (20–30%)	Weight change (20–30%)	Nervousness (10%)
Emotion/lability (20%)	Headaches (20%)	Decreased libido (5%)

oral medroxyprogesterone acetate 10 mg t.i.d. for periods of 45 to 60 days. Common progestational side effects are listed in Table 7-1 (3,4).

Progestins may also have a role in stabilizing the endometrium of patients who have required estrogen to decrease significant blood loss. Stabilization of the endometrium with cessation of bleeding allows an increase in hematocrit in anemic patients as well as creating an even endometrium that will be appropriately shed once the progestin is withdrawn. This type of initial regimen may then be followed by other medical pretreatment regimens, i.e., gonadotropin-releasing hormone (GnRH) agonists, danazol, or further progestins.

Oral Contraceptives

Like progestins, oral contraceptives are often used clinically to regulate and decrease the amount of menstrual flow. Previous studies have documented decreases of greater than 40% of pretreatment loss using reliable methods for quantification of menstrual blood loss (5). Current combined oral contraceptives contain progestins in all active hormonal days, and thus, there is a continual antagonism to the estrogen component. It is for this reason oral contraceptives were considered a reasonable pretreatment option.

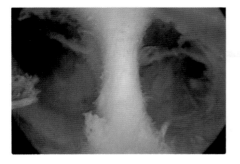

COLOR PLATE I

Hysteroscopic view of complete uterine septum.

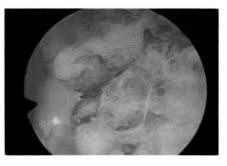

COLOR PLATE II

Resectoscopic resection of uterine septum with electric knife: initial division.

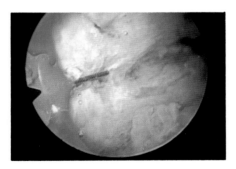

COLOR PLATE III

Resectoscopic resection of uterine septum with electric knife: deeper cutting.

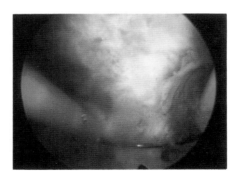

COLOR PLATE IV

Resectoscopic resection of uterine septum with 180° loop.

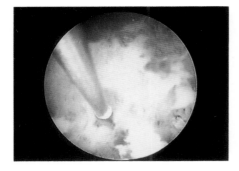

COLOR PLATE V

Hysteroscopic division of extensive fundal intrauterine adhesions: initial division of adhesions.

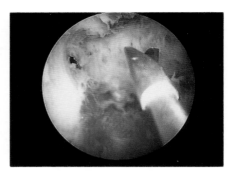

COLOR PLATE VI

Hysteroscopic division of extensive fundal intrauterine adhesions: right uterotubal cone is visible.

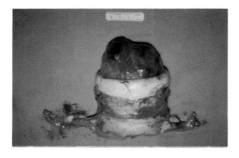

COLOR PLATE VII

The size of submucous myomas is probably self-limiting—this fibroid measuring approximately 6 cm could no longer be contained in the uterine cavity.

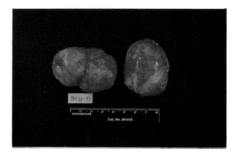

COLOR PLATE VIII

These leiomyomas, which were removed intact through an abdominal incision, show that the shape of leiomyomas is not always round. More may lie intramural than is apparent on hysteroscopic view. A grading scale would probably correctly have identified the degree of intramural extension for the leiomyoma on the right. However, the constricted area as seen on the specimen on the left could have given the impression that the intramural portion was smaller than that projecting into the uterine cavity.

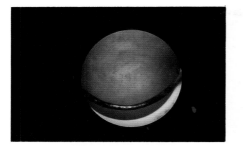

COLOR PLATE IX

The appearance of the uterine cavity at the start of endometrial resection.

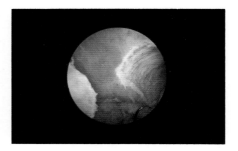

COLOR PLATE X

The endometrial/myometrial interface during surgery.

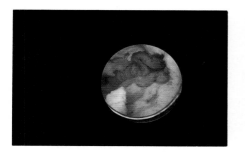

COLOR PLATE XI

The appearance of the uterine cavity at the end of endometrial resection.

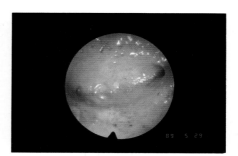

COLOR PLATE XII

Photo of uterus—normal cavity.

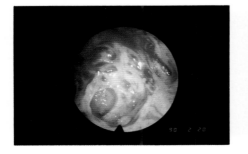

COLOR PLATE XIII

Photo of uterus—postablation (synechiae).

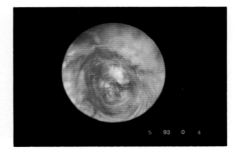

COLOR PLATE XIV

Photo of uterus—postablation (narrowed and cylindrical).

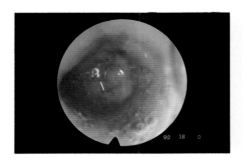

COLOR PLATE XV

Uterine cavity before curettage.

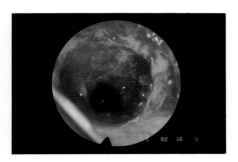

COLOR PLATE XVI

Uterine cavity after curettage.

Unfortunately, the estrogenic stimulus is not completely suppressed, even on very low-dose preparations. Because of this, there are relatively few patients who become amenorrheic from atrophy, and most patients have some level of endometrial proliferation. Although the endometrium is decreased compared to the ovulatory patient, there may be enough endometrium to interfere with visualization.

In the case of patients being pretreated prior to endometrial ablation, there may be difficulty in achieving destruction of the endometrium to the basal level. Previous publications have documented the ability of continuous oral contraceptives to cause a decidual-like effect and amenorrhea, thus the term *pseudo-pregnancy*. As with progestins, there is a variable response of the endometrium, and many months of treatment may be required to achieve the desired effect. It is for these reasons the authors have found limited utility for oral contraceptives in preoperative endometrial preparation for hysteroscopy.

Danazol

Danazol has been used extensively in Europe for preoperative endometrial preparation. Danazol is a 2,3-isoxazol derivative of 17(alpha)-ethinyl testosterone. The medication was introduced over two decades ago and has been studied as a treatment in numerous gynecologic disorders.

Pharmacodynamic studies have shown that the drug is almost completely absorbed from the GI tract with peak serum levels 2 hours later and almost no drug seen after 8 hours (6). It is from this data and efficacy data that the recommended regimen is 200 mg every 6 to 8 hours.

Danazol has multiple mechanisms of action. Baseline levels of gonadotropins are unchanged, but there is a decrease in mid-cycle gonadotropin surge. Estradiol levels are decreased to a low follicular phase level. Sex hormone-binding globulin levels are markedly decreased with a subsequent elevation in free testosterone levels. This explains the increased prevalence of androgenic symptoms in patients taking Danazol.

While recent studies have suggested comparable efficacy of lower doses and decreased side effects with the diminished dose, this is in disagreement with other trials (7,8). In addition, there is concern that decreased doses may not cause full suppression because of the metabolism of the drug, and this may, in turn, cause less endometrial suppression in the pretreatment patient. Unfortunately, as the clinician increases the dose, significant side effects are seen (Table 7-1).

In general, patients should be placed on medication for 6 weeks prior to undergoing surgery. In addition, an effort should be made to rule out pregnancy as the potential for virilization exists should pregnancy occur (9).

GnRH Agonists

GnRH agonists (GnRHa) were originally introduced as a medical treatment for patients with prostate cancer. In recent years, many applications for these agents to gynecologic disease have been evaluated. During initial animal trials, it was noted that acute administration of GnRHa caused a stimulatory effect, as would be expected for an agent with an agonist effect (10). Chronic administration, to the surprise of the investigators, caused pituitary downregulation and desensitization, acting in an almost antagonist fashion. Reversal of administration caused a return to the original stimulatory effect. This may be seen graphically in Figure 7-2. When given chronically, there is a variable period of agonist stimulation for 6 to 10 ($\pm$ 2) days. A period of decreased hypothalamic-pituitary-ovarian axis function follows with an eventual reversible senescence. Investigations have suggested several mechanisms by which this type of phenomenon might occur. It is hypothesized the receptor site/agonist complex causes downregulation and an uncoupling of the receptor/agonist occurs to cause a desensitization effect. The end result is a pseudo-menopausal state with very low levels of circulating estradiol. It is this effect that is most clinically useful in the preoperative preparation of patients.

GnRHa are synthesized by modifying the native GnRH molecule at the N-terminal end and near the sixth amino acid. These

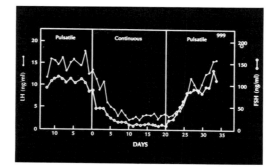

FIGURE 7-2

Pulsatile administration of GnRH in an ovariectomized monkey demonstrates normal gonadotropin release. Continuous infusion induces an incremental decrease over 7 to 10 days. Reinstitution of the intermittent or pulsatile release reverses the suppression with a return to baseline gonadotropin levels. Reproduced with permission from Belchetz PE, Plant TM, Nakai Y, Keogh EJ, Knobil E. Hypophysial responses to continuous and intermittent delivery of hypothalamic gonadotropin-releasing hormone. Science 1978;202:632.

chemical changes impart greater potency and inhibit degradation enzymes, thereby extending the half-life. Three GnRHa are presently approved in the United States for the treatment of endometriosis: nafarelin acetate, leuprolide acetate, and goserelin acetate. Table 7-2 summarizes the dosimetry for the various GnRHa available. All three have different delivery systems. Nafarelin is available as a 400-μg intranasal spray. Leuprolide is available in either a depoformulation of microspheres or as a subcutaneous daily injection and goserelin is available as a long-acting subcutaneous implant.

GnRHa have been shown to decrease the size of a significant percent of all fibroids, decrease uterine volume, and elevate hemoglobin levels during treatment. In a European multicenter study, Serra reported that treatment with four months of GnRHa resulted in 53% of individual myomas decreasing in size more than 50% of the inital pretreatment volume, while 18% of myomas were unchanged or increased in size (11). Friedman and colleagues found

TABLE 7-2

Commonly Used GnRH Analogs: Administration and Dosage*

GENERIC NAME	TRADE NAME	AVAILABLE IN U.S.	RATE OF ADMINISTRATION	DOSE
Leuprolide	Lupron	yes	IM	3.75–7.5 mg/monthly
			SQ	0.5–1.0 mg/daily
Nafarelin	Synarel	yes	Intranasal	400–800 μg/daily
Goserelin	Zoladex	yes	SQ implant	3.6 mg/monthly
Tryptorelin	Decapeptyl	no	IM	3.75 mg/monthly
			SQ	0.25–0.5 mg/daily
Buserelin	Suprefact	no	IM	Intramuscular 900–1200 μg/daily

SQ = subcutaneous.
*The three agonists available in the United States and two agonists commonly used outside the United States are compared for route of administration and dosing.

similar results in their randomized, prospective, double-blind multi-center study (12). They demonstrated a mean uterine volume reduction of 36% at 12 weeks and 45% at 24 weeks in patients treated with leuprolide acetate. It is from this data that most clinicians consider 3 months of pretreatment adequate to reduce myoma size. Shorter treatment regimens have also been evaluated. In one study, a short course GnRHa treatment regimen found a volume reduction of 35% at one month and 44% at 2 months (13).

Golan and coworkers evaluated the GnRHa D-Trp 6-LHRH and found a decrease in operative times and the amount of intraoperative blood loss (14).

In patients presenting with menorrhagia and anemia, immediate surgery may have a higher incidence of blood transfusion. Vercellini and colleagues demonstrated a mean hemoglobin rise from 8.5 to 13.3 g/dL in patients treated for 6 months with the GnRHa goserelin (15). Interestingly, 51% of their control group required blood transfusion whereas no medical treatment patient was transfused intra- or postoperatively.

Suction Curettage Prior to Hysteroscopy

Several reports have discussed the use of a suction curette to mechanically denude the endometrium prior to operative hysteroscopy. In these cases, preoperative medication is not required. Interestingly, one author felt performance of the procedure during the late luteal or menstrual phase of the cycle allowed the clearest visualization (16). He hypothesized that late luteal or menstrual endometrium may be more loosely attached and, thus, more easily separated from the basalis during suction. Performance of a procedure during these time periods does risk interruption of a chemically nondetectable pregnancy. In a second report, the procedure was performed during the early follicular phase without difficulty (17). Both authors felt the advantages of this type of preparation were (1) cost savings; (2) no wait for medication to cause endometrial atrophy; and (3) obtaining tissue for histologic evaluation. In one patient, preoperative endometrial biopsy demonstrated anovulatory endometrium without atypia. At the time of endometrial ablation, suction curettage demonstrated atypical hyperplasia. Concern was raised regarding the possible suppressive effect of a preoperative medication. The clinical relevance of abnormal endometrium that suppresses to normal is debatable. In addition, endometrial biopsies have demonstrated an impressive ability to rule out endometrial disease (18). However, regardless of the technique used for ablation and preparation, suspicious or unusual areas seen during precedures should be biopsied or resected for histologic analysis, regardless of previous histology.

EFFICACY OF PRETREATMENT REGIMENS

In DeCherney's original publication on the use of the urologic resectoscope to manage patients with septa, polyps, myomata, and abnormal uterine bleeding, no specific pretreatment regimen was utilized (1). Septum patients had surgery during the proliferative phase. Patients with intractable uterine bleeding had all been initially treated with 25 mg of IV conjugated estrogens and failed. They then underwent endometrial cauterization using the wire loop.

In 1989, Vancaillie reported on the use of a ball-end resectoscope to ablate the endometrium in 15 patients (19). He suggested that menstruation might be the ideal period in which to perform ablation, but dismissed this as "technically difficult." His regimen of pre-treatment was daily oral medroxyprogesterone acetate, 5 mg/75 lb, beginning on day 2 of the cycle with performance of the procedure 3 to 4 weeks later. In short-term follow-up, 14 of 15 patients had amenorrhea or hypomenorrhea.

Goldrath reported on the use of danazol for treatment prior to laser endometrial ablation (20). He recommended 800 mg/day for 25 days prior to surgery and described a "very thin atrophic endometrium in which telangiectasia is present." Using this proto-col, he had excellent or good results in 299 of 321 women.

In contrast to Goldrath, Lefler and colleagues reported about patients undergoing endometrial coagulation: ". . . Danazol re-sulted in inconsistent thinning of the endometrium which often shredded off, obscuring vision during the procedure, and which may have left thicker areas of the endometrium uncoagulated" (17). They reported a nonstatistically significant increase in amenorrhea rates in patients who underwent coagulation ablation using vaso-pressin and suction curettage versus patients undergoing laser abla-tion and a pretreatment regimen of 200 mg of danazol twice daily.

Gimpelson and Kaigh compared results obtained with a hetero-geneous group of medical preparations (danazol, leuprolide, and nafarelin) to patients who underwent suction curettage prior to endo-metrial ablation (16). Their study was neither prospective nor ran-domized but offered interesting conclusions. No statistical differ-ences were noted between the study groups when evaluating for reduction of bleeding or amenorrhea. Nonstatistically significant de-creases in operative times and the amount of fluids used or absorbed were seen in the suction curettage group. Because the suction curet-tage patients were later in the series, influence of operator experience and equipment evolution make comparisons difficult. This form of pretreatment offers the theoretic advantages of decreased cost and additional histologic specimen. Some surgeons have suggested the addition of a procedure (suction curettage) might lead to increased operative times and, thus, the question of increasing operating room cost. In addition, there are concerns regarding the ability of suction curettage to completely denude the endometrium to the level of the basalis to allow the most effective destruction when performing endometrial coagulation. Such issues may be less important when performing endometrial resection (see Chapter 12). It is also difficult to understand how suction curettage, which causes endometrial trauma and bleeding, would lead to decreased intravasation from these open vessels.

While additional tissue may be sent for further histologic evaluation, it is the editor's recommendation that all patients being considered for ablative procedures be adequately evaluated prior to ablation with office sampling, hysteroscopy, or previous dilatation/curettage. While one patient was documented to have abnormal histology at the time of ablation (which was normal at previous sampling), it is unclear how such abnormalities might respond to medical pretreatment. Randomized, prospective evaluations may help in answering these critical questions.

Brooks and Serden reported on the use of a single dose of the GnRHa leuprolide acetate depot prior to resectoscopic endometrial ablation (21). When administered during the luteal phase, the agonist effect is generally inconsequential. Following menses, pituitary downregulation and desensitization will have occurred. At this point, endogenous estradiol levels should be close to castrate, and little proliferation should occur in the postmenstrual basal endometrium. Interestingly, anecdotal reports have described increased bleeding in either preablation or myomectomy patients following GnRHa administration. Although relatively uncommon, expectant hormonal management with estrogen is appropriate in these cases, and rarely is surgical treatment necessary. In patients treated with a single dose of GnRHa, Brooks described the endometrium as being ". . . thinned in all patients, with inactive glands, reduced vascularity, and atrophic stroma."

Serden and Brooks compared amenorrhea rates achieved following ablation with either no preparation, danazol, progestins, or leuprolide acetate (22). Progesterones were dropped from the protocol because of the difficulties with tissue from the decidualized endometrium interfering with surgery. Amenorrhea rates were 41% for danazol, 43% with no preparation, and 67% for leuprolide acetate during the short follow-up. In another study, various preoperative treatment strategies were compared by analyzing the endometrial histology from the resected tissue (23). Progestins (DMPA or norethindrone) were noted to induce endometrial thickening secondary to tissue edema. Vascular proliferation and angiectasia were noted with this preparation (Figure 7-3). In patients who were untreated but had their surgery performed during the proliferative phase, the endometrium was described as thin and hypovascular but histologically dysfunctional. Patients treated with depo-leuprolide acetate had reproducible results, with the endometrium noted to be

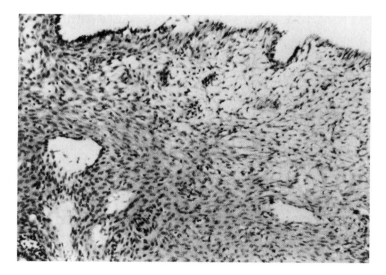

FIGURE 7-3

Photomicrograph of endometrium after progestin therapy. Edema, angiectasia, and decidual reaction are notable. Reproduced with permission from Brooks PG, Serden SP, Davos I. Hormonal inhibition of the endometrium for resectoscopic endometrial ablation. Am J Obstet Gynecol 1991;164:1602.

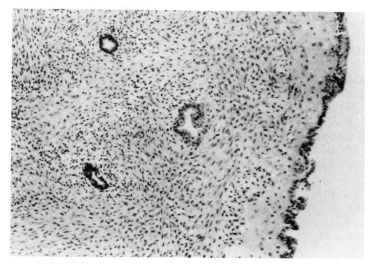

FIGURE 7-4

Photomicrograph of endometrium after leuprolide therapy, showing atrophy, sparse glands, and dense stroma. Reproduced with permission from Brooks PG, Serden SP, Davos I. Hormonal ablation. Am J Obstet Gynecol 1991;164:1602.

thin, mostly atrophic, and without tissue edema (Figure 7-4). In contrast, Danazol demonstrated a variable effect, which was reported to be independent of dose or duration of treatment. The endometrium was found to be dysynchronous with variable vascularity and tissue thickness (Figure 7-5).

In another study evaluating efficiency of GnRHa, Perino and colleagues prospectively compared leuprolide acetate to no treatment in patients undergoing septal incision, endometrial ablation, and submucous myomectomy (24). They documented no difference in the septum group but found statistically significant reductions in operative time, intraoperative bleeding, volume of media infused, and failure rates (continued abnormal bleeding after 1 year or persistence of fibroid after 2 months) in the group of patients undergoing submucous myomectomy and pretreated with a GnRHa. In the endometrial ablation pretreatment group, decreases were seen in

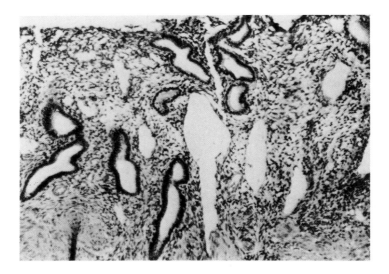

FIGURE 7-5

Photomicrograph of endometrium after danazol therapy. Angiectasia is extensive and thickness is less than with progestins. Reproduced with the permission from Brooks PG, Serden SP, Davos I. Hormonal inhibition of the endometrium for resectoscopic endometrial ablation. Am J Obstet Gynecol 1991;164:1602.

operative time, intraoperative bleeding and media used, but similar failure rates were recorded.

The choice of a pretreatment regimen depends on physician preference and skill, type of procedure to be performed, and preoperative status, i.e., hemoglobin. Many authors have "favorite" protocols; the editor's standard pretreatment regimens are presented in Table 7-3.

POSTOPERATIVE TREATMENT

Postoperative endometrial suppression has gained increasing interest as clinicians strive to achieve higher amenorrhea rates. The idea of postoperative suppression is based on the premise that many women will have islands of noncoagulated or partially coagulated

TABLE 7-3

Pretreatment Protocols for Endometrial and
Myoma Preparation

Surgical Procedure	Pretreatment Regimen*
Endometrial ablation	GnRHa × 2 months (if begun follicular phase) GnRHa × 1 to 2 months (if begun luteal phase)
Septum resection	Surgery during proliferative phase or luteal phase GnRHa
Endometrial resection	Surgery during proliferative phase or GnRHa agonist × 1 to 2 months
Myomectomy	GnRHa × 3 months (depending on size)
Polypectomy	No pretreatment

*Pretreatment regimens will vary depending on the clinical scenario. This table gives the editors' most commonly used protocols for endometrial and myoma preparation.

endometrium that will ultimately regenerate and lead to menstrual bleeding. In many cases, there is likely to be residual endometrium as 50% of women continue to have some level of bleeding following ablation. Some clinicians believe that postoperative hormonal inhibition will decrease the stimulus for regeneration of such tissues, possibly improving the overall success rate. Townsend and colleagues used such a regimen when they first reported on rollerball coagulation (25). Twenty-five of 50 patients treated received 400 mg of medroxyprogesterone in the recovery room. None of these patients had bleeding in a follow-up period of 6 to 12 months. Unfortunately, their long-term follow-up was not published.

In one of the only published reports addressing this issue, Goldrath found a significant improvement in amenorrhea rates after Nd-YAG laser ablation and a postoperative injection of 150 mg of medroxyprogesterone acetate (20). The group of patients treated

with ablation alone without postoperative treatment had an amenorrhea rate of 37.3%, whereas those treated with both ablation and
postoperative DMPA had a 69.3% rate of amenorrhea. The overall
success rate (nonpersistence of menorrhagia) was similar in both
groups, but the increase in amenorrhea in the treatment group was
impressive. Unfortunately, the groups are not compared as to
length of time from surgery to re-evaluation, nor is comment made
as to when cases were performed relative to the author's experience.
Goldrath additionally alludes to the use of Danocrine postoperatively but dismisses this as impractical because of the extended healing period (up to 6 months) for the endometrium.

GnRHa have also been suggested as post-treatment adjuvants.
It is felt that the significant hypoestrogenism these agents produce
may also retard or prevent regeneration of damaged tissue. Although studies are currently evaluating these agents, no published
studies are available.

Caustic agents, such as tetracyline, have also been considered for
postoperative treatment (personal communication, Vancaillie). It is
proposed that intrauterine installation of these compounds may also
serve to inhibit further tissue regeneration or proliferation. Concerns
include the risk of transtubal leakage into the peritoneal cavity, intravasation of the material, and vaginal irritation following installation.
As with the other proposed medical regimens, significant data is
lacking regarding efficacy and incidence of potential complications.

Because of our clinical desire to achieve higher amenorrhea
rates, we have become increasingly interested in managing the postoperative period. Unfortunately, the paucity of data does not aid in
choosing a regimen. Consideration must be given to the side effects,
cost, and potential risks of any medication used postoperatively.

CLINICAL PEARLS

✖ Diagnostic hysteroscopy is best performed during
the early proliferative phase.

✖ Progestational agents are useful in antagonizing the
effects of estrogen and in limiting endometrial growth.

✖ Danazol is a testosterone derivative that has many effects, including decreasing the midcycle gonadotropin surge and reducing estradiol levels to low follicular phase.

✖ GnRHa initially cause a gonadotropin surge with estrogen release but, with chronic administration, reduce gonadotropins and decrease estradiol to menopausal levels.

✖ GnRHa have been extensively used to decrease myoma size and vascularity and elevate hemoglobin prior to surgery.

✖ Few good studies exist comparing the efficacy of different regimens.

✖ Preliminary data suggest thinner endometrium allows better visualization and may have higher success rates with decreased intravasation because of decreased vascularity.

✖ Progestins cause a decidual-like effect that may interfere with operative hysteroscopy.

✖ Post-treatment regimens are being evaluated in an attempt to increase amenorrhea and overall success rates.

REFERENCES

1. DeCherney A, Polan ML. Hysteroscopic management of intrauterine lesions and intractable uterine bleeding. Obstet Gynecol 1983;61: 392–396.
2. Ortiz A, Hiroi M, Stanczyk F, et al. Serum medroxyprogesterone acetate (MPA) concentrations and ovarian function following intramuscular injection of depo-MPA. J Clin Endocrinol Metab 1977;44: 32–38.
3. Schwallie PC, Assenzo JR. Contraceptive use efficacy study utilizing medroxyprogesterone acetate administered as an intramuscular injection once every 90 days. Fertil Steril 1993;24:331–339.

4. Physicians Desk Reference, 48th ed. Oradell, NJ: Medical Economic Co., 1994:2442–2443.

5. Nilsson L, Rybo G. Treatment of menorrhagia. Am J Obstet Gynecol 1971;110:713–720.

6. Israel R. Pelvic endometriosis. In: Mishell DR, Davajan V, Lobo RA, eds. Infertility, contraception, and reproductive endocrinology. Boston: Blackwell Scientific Publications, 1991:734–735.

7. Biberoglu KO, Behrman SJ. Dosage aspects of danazol therapy in endometriosis: short-term and long-term effectiveness. Am J Obstet Gynecol 1981;139:645–654.

8. Dmowski WP, Kapetanakis E, Scommegna A. Variable effects of danazol on endometriosis at 4 low-dose levels. Obstet Gynecol 1982;59:408–415.

9. Quagliarello J, Greco MA. Danazol and urogenital sinus formation in pregnancy. Fertil Steril 1985;43:939–942.

10. Belchetz PE, Plant TM, Nakai Y, Keogh EJ, Knobil E. Hypophysial responses to continuous and intermittent delivery of hypothalamic gonadotropin-releasing hormone. Science 1978;202:631–633.

11. Serra GB, Panetta V, Colosimo M, et al. Efficacy of leuprolide acetate depot in symptomatic fibromatous uteri: the Italian multicentre trial. Clin Ther 1992;14:57–73.

12. Friedman AJ, Hoffman DI, Comite F, Browneller RW, Miller JD. Treatment of leiomyomata uteri with leuprolide acetate depot—a double-blind, placebo controlled multicenter study. Obstet Gynecol 1991;77:720–725.

13. Coddington CC, Brzyski R, Hansen KA, Corley DR, McIntyre-Seltman K, Jones HW. Short-term treatment with leuprolide acetate is a successful adjunct to surgical therapy of leiomyomas of the uterus. Surg Gynecol Obstet 1992;175:57–63.

14. Golan A, Bukovsky I, Pansky M, Schneider D, Weinraub Z, Caspi E. Preoperative gonadotropin-releasing hormone agonist treatment in surgery for uterine leiomyomata. Hum Reprod 1993;8:450–452.

15. Vercellini P, Bocciolone L, Columbo A, et al. Gonadotropin-releasing hormone agonist treatment before hyperectomy for menorrhagia and uterine leiomyomas. Acta Obstet Gynecol Scand 1993;72:369–373.

16. Gimpelson RJ, Kaigh J. Mechanical preparation of the endometrium prior to endometrial ablation. J Reprod Med 1992;37:691–694.

17. Lefler HT, Sullivan GH, Hulka JF. Modified endometrial ablation:

electrocoagulation with vasopressin and suction curettage preparation. Obstet Gynecol 1991;77:949–953.

18. Goldschmit R, Katz Z, Blickstein I, Caspi B, Dqaui R. The accuracy of endometrial pipette sampling with and without sonographic measurement of endometrium. Obstet Gynecol 1993;82:727–730.

19. Vancaillie TG. Electrocoagulation of the endometrium with the ball-end resectoscope. Obstet Gynecol 1989;74:425–427.

20. Goldrath MH. Use of danazol in hysteroscopic surgery for menorrhagia. J Reprod Med 1990;35:91–95.

21. Brooks PG, Serden SP. Preparation of the endometrium for ablation with a single dose of leuprolide acetate depot. J Reprod Med 1991;36:477–478.

22. Serden SP, Brooks PG. Preoperative therapy in preparation for endometrial ablation. J Reprod Med 1992;37:679–681.

23. Brooks PG, Serden SP, Davos I. Hormonal inhibition of the endometrium for resectoscopic endometrial ablation. Am J Obstet Gynecol 1991;164:1601–1606.

24. Perino A, Chianchiano N, Petronio M, Cittadini E. Role of leuprolide acetate depot in hysteroscopic surgery: a controlled study. Fertil Steril 1993;59:507–510.

25. Townsend DE, Richart RM, Paskowith RA, Woolfork RE. "Rollerball" coagulation of the endometrium. Obstet Gynecol 1990;76:310–313.

8

Uterine Septa

Rafael F. Valle

S eptate uterus distorts the symmetry of the uterine cavity and may interfere with normal reproduction. When surgical treatment is required, it can be provided transcervically via the hysteroscope utilizing a variety of mechanical methods. These include thermal energies via the resectoscope and laser energy via fiberoptic lasers.

EMBRYOLOGY AND ANATOMY

The fallopian tubes and the uterus are of Müllerian origin; in early embryologic development, the paramesonephric ducts fuse caudally and distally to form the upper vagina and the uterus while the remaining upper segments result in the fallopian tubes. This process begins at 4 to 6 weeks of embryologic life and usually is completed at 12 to 14 weeks of gestational age. In the absence of Müllerian inhibiting factor (MIF) produced by the testes, the paramesonephric or Müllerian ducts will progress to normal development. The uterine septum usually completes its reabsorption by 19 to 20 weeks of embryologic life. Failure to reabsorb will result in a septate uterus with partial or complete septation (1).

The anatomy resulting from arrest at fusion, cannalization, or reabsorption will depend upon the degree and stage at which the arrest occurs. Because there is no failure of fusion with the septate uterus, the uterine body is uniform externally, differentiating this anomaly from the bicornuate uterus, in which there is lack of fusion, and an external division remains.

The septation of the uterine body encompasses various lengths and widths of the septum. While some septa are thin, others are broad and produce thinner and smaller uterine cavities. Some only partially divide the uterine cavity and others extend the entire length of the uterine corpus and, occasionally, the entire length of the uterine cervix. In 20 to 25% of these patients, concomitant septation of the vagina occurs; occasionally, bicornuate uteri have an additional septation of the uterus (2) (Figure 8-1).

INDICATIONS FOR TREATMENT

The majority of women with uterine septa reproduce successfully; only 20 to 25% suffer pregnancy wastage—usually late first trimester or early second trimester miscarriages initiated by minilabors and bleeding.

The relationship between the septate uterus and infertility remains controversial; the consensus is that this type of uterine anomaly does not cause infertility. Nonetheless, as the therapeutic approach to this anomaly has evolved, patients with primary infertility requiring assisted reproductive technologies or difficult treatments for infertility have been considered candidates for treatment of the uterine septation.

Since the presence of a uterine septum may not be the basis of a reproductive problem, preoperative evaluation is important. The hysterosalpingogram is the most accurate and effective method of diagnosing the septate uterus, particularly division of the uterine cavity. Nonetheless, it is important to evaluate other factors that may cause pregnancy wastage before deciding on surgical treatment of the uterine septum. A karyotype should be performed in both husband and wife, and a normal maturation of the endometrium should be evaluated with a late luteal phase endometrial biopsy and

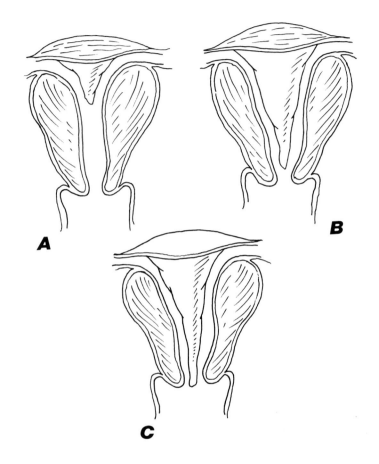

FIGURE 8-1

Diagrammatic representation of uterine septum: (a) partial uterine septum; (b) complete uterine septum; (c) complete septum with septate cervix.

a midluteal phase serum progesterone. Endocrine conditions, such as hypothyroidism, should be evaluated with a thyroid-stimulating hormone (TSH) assay.

Autoimmune and alloimmune conditions must be ruled out with a lupus anticoagulant factor study and partial thromboplastin time (PTT), as well as anticardiolipin antibodies (ACA) and antinuclear antibodies (ANA). Chronic endometritis is best ruled out with endometrial biopsy.

Finally, because of the close embryologic relationship of Müllerian structures to the mesonephric ducts, when these anomalies occur, renal anomalies should be ruled out. Although these urinary tract anomalies are not as marked and frequent with the septate uterus, duplication of calyceal systems, renal ptosis, and other such anomalies have been described. Therefore, it is valuable to evaluate these patients with a screening intravenous pyelogram (IVP) (3,4).

METHODS OF TREATMENT

In the past, invasive surgical treatments requiring laparotomy and hysterotomy were performed only in habitual aborters—women experiencing more than three spontaneous miscarriages in the early or mid-second trimester of pregnancy. With new, less invasive approaches, such as hysteroscopic treatment, the indications have been liberalized to focus the attention on each individual patient and her unique reproductive failure (5).

Until the introduction of the hysteroscopic approach, the surgical treatment of the symptomatic uterine septum was by abdominal metroplasty of the Jones or Tompkins type.

The Jones abdominal metroplasty involves the transfundal excision of the septum by removing a cuneiform portion of the fundal myometrium with subsequent surgical repair (6). This technique has resulted in over 80% viable pregnancies and has been used as the standard for success of procedures to correct the symptomatic septate uterus. Disadvantages with this procedure are the need for laparotomy, hysterotomy, and the possibility of postoperative adhesions, particularly at the tubal ovarian regions, sometimes resulting in secondary infertility. Once the patient has a hysterotomy, the waiting period before attempting pregnancy is prolonged (3 to 6 months). Should a pregnancy occur and be carried to term, a cesarean section is mandatory.

The Tompkins procedure involves bisection of the uterus in the anteroposterior plane and transverse division of the uterine septum without excision of myometrial tissue (7). This technique bleeds less than the Jones procedure and results in a more uniform uterine cavity that is not reduced in size. For this reason, most practitioners prefer the second approach to treat the septate uterus. Nonetheless, hysterotomy carries the disadvantage of the need for a 3- to 6-month waiting period until pregnancy is permitted. A cesarean section is required when the pregnancy is carried to term to prevent possible uterine dehiscence.

HYSTEROSCOPIC METROPLASTY

Hysteroscopic treatment provides a less invasive approach to divide the uterine septum. In a hysteroscopic approach, as with the abdominal metroplasty of the Tompkins type, the septum is divided under direct vision, the avascular consistency of this embryologic remnant inhibiting significant bleeding. Resection of the septum is not necessary as the septal remnants are pulled into the uterine musculature. The hysteroscopic approach permits this condition to be treated as an ambulatory procedure with minimal discomfort to the patient as well as minimal morbidity (8–12). Because the uterine wall is not invaded, a cesarean section is required only for obstetrical indications. The healing process with re-epithelialization of the uterine cavity takes only 4 to 5 weeks, so patients are allowed to conceive sooner than with abdominal metroplasty. Hospitalization is not required, so expenses are markedly reduced.

There are three different approaches to the hysteroscopic metroplasty (Figure 8-2): mechanical division with hysteroscopic scissors; resectoscopic division with electrosurgery; and fiberoptic laser division of the uterine septum.

Hysteroscopic Metroplasty with Scissors

Hysteroscopic metroplasty with scissors is the most common method used. An operative hysteroscope with a 7 French operative channel is

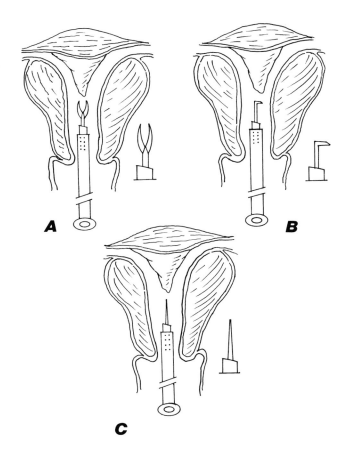

FIGURE 8-2

Hysteroscopic metroplasty: (a) scissors; (b) resectoscope; (c) fiberoptic laser.

required. A continuous flow system to monitor fluids infused and recovered is ideal to monitor nonrecovered fluid and prevent excessive intravasation. Hysteroscopic scissors can be flexible, semirigid, or rigid. The flexible scissors are difficult to manipulate. Semirigid scissors are most commonly used as they permit a targeted division of the tissue, they can be selectively directed to the area in need of dissection, and they can be retrieved at will when a better panoramic view is required. The semirigid scissors can be directed easily without much force or manipulation through the operating channel of the hysteroscope, facilitating hysteroscopic surgery, but they must be sharpened and tightened frequently. Scissors of the hook type are most helpful to divide the uterine septum, particularly when reaching the broad fundal area where small superficial cuts must be made on the remaining septum to sculpture this fundal area and avoid deep penetration (Figures 8-3, 8-4 and 8-5).

The rigid scissors, often called optical scissors and fixed to the end of the hysteroscope, can also be used to divide fibrotic and broad septa. When using the fixed instrument, it is important to have a perfect panoramic view while performing the division. The scissors should be introduced with utmost care to avoid uterine

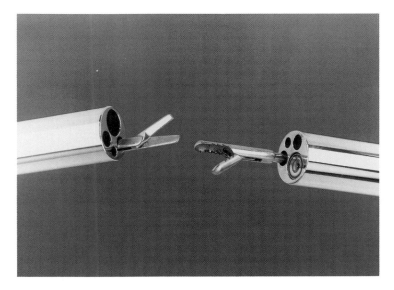

FIGURE 8-3

Weck-Baggish hysteroscopy with double operating channels (scissors on left, grasping forceps on right).

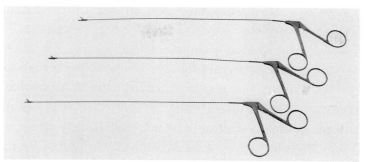

FIGURE 8-4

Semirigid hysteroscopic instruments.

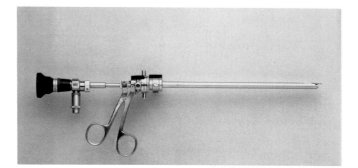

FIGURE 8-5

Operating hysteroscope (Olympus) with rigid fixed scissors in place.

damage as their sharp tips can easily perforate the uterus if force is exerted against the uterine wall.

With the use of mechanical tools in operative hysteroscopy, the best medium to distend the uterine cavity is one that contains electrolytes, particularly sodium (Na), permitting more volume to be intravasated during a procedure without the development of hyponatremia. Normal saline, dextrose 5% in half normal saline (D_5 0.45% NaCl), or Ringer's lactate, a balanced solution, can be safely used with good visualization properties.

The technique of uterine septal division with hysteroscopic scissors involves dividing the septum exactly at the midline, where tissue is more fibrotic and avascular. The novice approaching this operation tends to drift to the posterior uterine wall in an anterior uterus or the anterior wall in a posterior uterus. When this occurs, the vessels may reach the septum from the myometrial tissue, causing unnecessary bleeding. The division is performed systematically from side to side, cutting small portions of the septum with each bite. Once the uterotubal cones are visualized, the cuts become more shallow and the small vessels crossing the septum from the myometrium should be closely observed to avoid penetrating the myometrial tissue. With the laparoscope in place and the light dimmed, an assistant observes the translucency of the hysteroscopic light through the uterine wall, warning the hysteroscopist of any increase in translucency as the division progresses in this fundal area. Once the septal division is completed, and before the instruments are removed, the uterine fundal area is observed hysteroscopically while decreasing the intrauterine pressure. This is done to observe significant bleeding. In the presence of arterial bleeding, selective coagulation is performed (Figure 8-6).

There are several advantages of dividing the uterine septum with scissors (Table 8-1). This simple technique can be performed quickly and is applicable to practically all septa. The scissors can easily be guided into the recessed areas of the septum. Because no electricity is used, the media to distend the uterine cavity may contain electrolytes. This gives a safety margin for utilization of fluids since more volume may be used as compared with fluids devoid of electrolytes. Finally, no additional expense of energy is required.

There are a few disadvantages to using this technique. Small scissors can become easily dulled and loose and may not cut precisely, so they should be exchanged periodically and repaired. Also, if division of the septum is not maintained in the midline, bleeding may occur. Sharp scissors may cause perforation if not controlled in

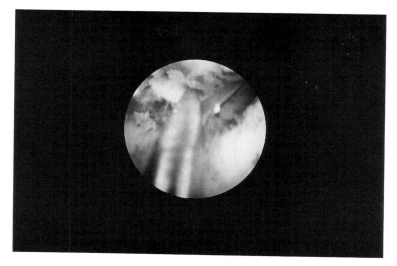

FIGURE 8-6

Hysteroscopic division of partial uterine septum.

TABLE 8-1

Hysteroscopic Division of Uterine Septa (Scissors)

Advantages	Disadvantages
Simple	Scissors get dull
Quick	Bleeding if not in midline
Applicable to all septa	Possible perforation
Media with electrolytes	No washing effect unless
No energy sources required	double channel hysteroscope used

the uterine fundal and cornual regions. Finally, not all hysteroscopes have perfect continuous flow; therefore, a washing effect cannot be provided unless a double channel hysteroscope is available.

Resectoscopic Division of the Uterine Septum

Resectoscopic division of the uterine septum provides hemostasis if a true midline incision is not maintained but may involve more lateral tissue destruction. A gynecologic resectoscope, 8 to 9 mm outer diameter, with a narrow and thin electrode (cutting loop, preferably pointed forward, knife electrode or wire electrode), can be used to divide the septum by contact electrosurgery. Knives and electrodes have been modified for this purpose and are available from the various manufacturing companies. Whether they are thinner or thicker depends upon the thickness of the tissue to be divided. The resectoscope allows a perfect continuous flow system that permits exact measurement of the volume of fluid infused and recovered and provides continuous washing of the uterine cavity and a clear view, removing bubbles and debris during the procedure (Figures 8-7 to 8-10).

Because electricity is used with the resectoscope, only fluids devoid of electrolytes can be utilized (see Chapter 5). A specific amount of nonrecovered fluid must be maintained during the procedure because excessive fluid intravasation can occur, causing fluid overload that is worsened by the lack of electrolytes and results in hyponatremia.

The uterine septum is divided, beginning at its apex or nadir, by short and brief contacts of the loop or knife with the septum. This is the only time the resectoscope is used cutting forward rather

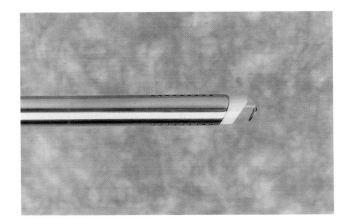

FIGURE 8-7

Distal end of resectoscope (Storz) with resecting loop in place.

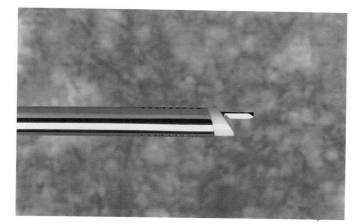

FIGURE 8-8

Distal end of resectoscope (Storz) with knife electrode.

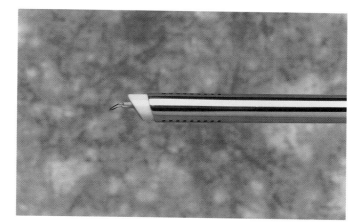

FIGURE 8-9

Distal end of resectoscope (Storz) with forward-cutting loop.

than with the shaving motion toward the operator commonly used in polyp, myoma, or endometrial resection. Extra care should be used in determining the exact depth of penetration and direction of the electrode. Laparoscopic monitoring is mandatory. It is important to observe the symmetry of both uterotubal cones and, with

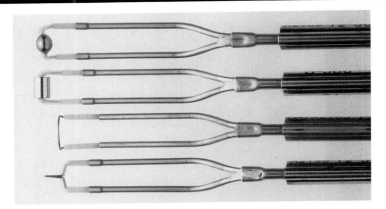

FIGURE 8-10

Electrodes for use with resectoscope. Top to bottom: rollerball, rollerbar, resecting loop, cutting knife (Olympus).

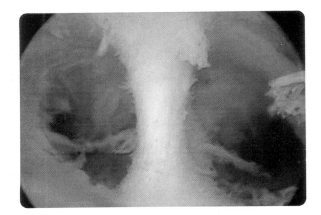

FIGURE 8-11

Hysteroscopic view of complete uterine septum.

laparoscopy, the transillumination the resectoscope's light produces through the uterine wall. The resectoscopic electrode will coagulate any vessel encountered, so upon reaching the fundal area, it is of utmost importance to avoid resection into the myometrial tissue. The contact of the electrode should become even more superficial and the resectoscopic transillumination more clearly observed by the assistant (Figures 8-11 to 8-13).

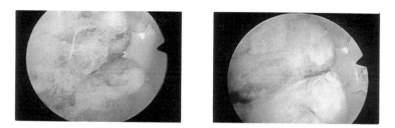

FIGURE 8-12

Resectoscopic resection of uterine septum with electric knife: (a) initial division; (b) deeper cutting.

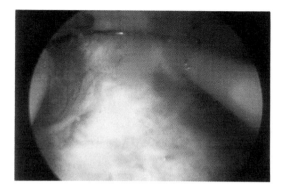

FIGURE 8-13

Resectoscopic resection of uterine septum with 180° loop.

While performing the division of the uterine septum utilizing electrosurgery, it is important to observe periodically from a distance the uterine cavity symmetry at the level of the internal os. During the division of the septum, this symmetry may not be evident while working close to the tissue.

With resectoscopic division of the uterine septum, bleeding is decreased; owing to the coagulating effect of the electrical energy, the cuts are easy and the uterine cavity is washed by the continuous flow of distending fluid through the resectoscope (13,14). Visualization is excellent and manipulation is easy.

The disadvantages are that monopolar electrical current is necessary and peripheral coagulation of the adjacent normal endometrium, a reservoir for future re-epithelialization of the area, may occur. Furthermore, at the juxtaposed myometrium, the landmarks are lost because the coagulating power of the electrical energy may not allow for observation of the small arterial bleeders usually observed with mechanical division.

The fluids used for these procedures cannot contain electrolytes in order to permit electrosurgery. Therefore, care must be taken to avoid hyponatremia if excessive intravasation occurs. Occasionally, a broad septum may make manipulation of the resectoscope difficult and these septa may be difficult to divide with the resectoscope (Table 8-2).

Hysteroscopic Metroplasty with Fiberoptic Lasers

Hysteroscopic metroplasty with fiberoptic lasers is similar in many ways to the resectoscopic methods. The septum can be divided with fiberoptic lasers, particularly the Nd-YAG with an extruded or sculptured fiber of the sharp type to permit cutting. The Argon or KTP-532 can also be used in this manner, although the lower power produced by these lasers makes the cutting more tedious. Extruded fibers are usually used in the uterus. Coaxial fibers with sapphire tips need to be cooled continuously, either by fluids or by gases. Fluid coolant may be used, but gases should never be used in the uterus to cool the sapphire tips because of the high flow

---

TABLE 8-2

Hysteroscopic Division of Uterine Septa (Resectoscope)

Advantages	Disadvantages
No bleeding	Electrosurgery required (monopolar)
Cuts easily	Possible lateral coagulation
Washing of uterine cavity	Landmarks of myometrium lost
Excellent visibility	Fluids without electrolytes
Easy manipulation	Difficult to divide broad septa

required of about 1 L per minute (Figures 8-14, 8-15). Because lasers are not conductive, electrolyte-containing fluids should be used to distend the uterine cavity. Normal saline, dextrose 5% in normal saline, or Ringer's lactate is most useful to distend the uterine cavity and obtain clear visualization. It is important to have some outflow with these hysteroscopic techniques to remove the debris and bubbles produced with the activated laser; therefore, a continuous flow hysteroscope or one with inflow and outflow channels is most advantageous.

Division of the uterine septum should begin at the nadir of the septum in the midline, dividing the septum from side to side. Care must be taken to move the fiber continuously to prevent boring into one hole. Because division of the septum with fiberoptic lasers may be somewhat tedious, the division should be systematic from side to side. The same precautions should be used as with division of the septum with electrocoagulation. Avoid invading the juxtaposed

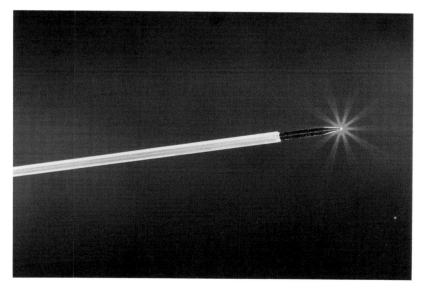

FIGURE 8-14

Quartz sculpted conical fiber for contact precise cutting and coagulating. (Tip size, 300 μ) (Laser Sonics).

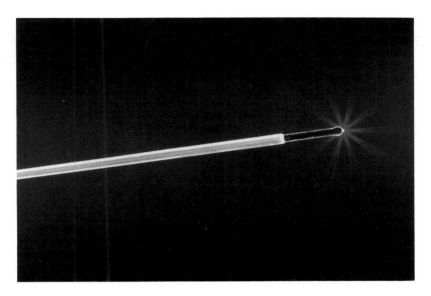

FIGURE 8-15

Quartz sculpted ball–shaped tip fiber for enhanced coagulation (Tip size, 1200µ) (Laser Sonics).

fundal myometrium as the coagulating power of the laser will also seal small arterial vessels at the fundal uterine wall.

There are advantages of the hysteroscopic division with fiberoptic lasers. Bleeding is avoided because of the coagulating power of the laser. This energy source cuts well and is easy to manipulate, perhaps even more easily manipulated than the resectoscope. Since there is a lack of conductivity, fluids with electrolytes can be used.

However, there are disadvantages. The laser is an expensive energy source and needs special protective glasses. Back-scattering of these fiberoptic lasers can damage the retina. The possibility of lateral scattering makes lasers potentially damaging to the normal endometrium peripheral to the septum. Damage of this peripheral endometrium may slow epithelialization of the newly denuded area (15). Finally, lasers require special maintenance and assistants, including a laser safety officer for operating the unit and appropriate eye protection for the assisting personnel.

TABLE 8-3

Hysteroscopic Division of Uterine Septa (Fiberoptic Lasers)

ADVANTAGES	DISADVANTAGES
No bleeding	Expensive
Cut well	Special protective glasses needed
Easy manipulation	Possible lateral scattering
Fluids with electrolytes	Require special maintenance and assistance (Laser safety officer)

Because the procedure may be tedious, excessive amounts of fluids may be required (16). Should the hysteroscope lack continuous flow system or a double channel to collect the returning fluid after cleansing the cavity from bubbles and debris, excessive fluid may be intravasated. In the absence of a perfect monitoring system for the inflow and outflow, the intravasated fluid may not be adequately measured, thereby endangering the patient with pulmonary edema secondary to fluid overload, despite the use of fluids with electrolytes. Therefore, it is important to monitor the fluid infused and maintain the intrauterine pressure so as not to exceed the mean arterial pressure of about 100 mmHg (17) (Table 8-3).

INTRAOPERATIVE AND POSTOPERATIVE MANAGEMENT

Prophylactic antibiotics are commonly used to prevent infection to the uterine cavity, and specifically to the fallopian tubes, when intrauterine manipulation is required. Intravenous cephalosporins can be used intraoperatively and continued for 3 to 4 days postoperatively in an oral form. Kefzol 1 mg IV piggyback is used half an hour prior to surgery, followed by Keflex 500 mg q.i.d. PO for 3 or 4 days following the procedure. While the use of high doses of estrogens, such as Premarin, is controversial, this medication may allow better and faster re-epithelialization of the denuded area left by the division of the septum. High doses, such as Premarin 2.5 mg b.i.d. PO for 30 days can be used and terminal progesterone added in the form of Provera 10 mg each day in the last 10 days of this artificial cycle. Once the patient completes withdrawal bleeding from hormonal therapy, a hysterosalpingogram can be performed to assess the symmetry of the uterine cavity. The woman may attempt pregnancy when a satisfactory result is obtained. Because of the axis by which the uterine cavity is observed, hysterosalpingography becomes an excellent method to assess the surgical results. Hysteroscopy, which looks for symmetry from the cervical axis, may provide an alternative appraisal of the uterine fundus. Either method can be utilized as long as the practitioner is aware of the drawbacks. It is not unusual to see a small central fundal residual septal projection on hysterosalpingography following hysteroscopic division of the uterine septum. Nonetheless, when a small residual septum less than 1 cm in length is observed, no additional therapy is performed, as this residual septum has no clinical significance.

RESULTS

The reproductive outcome following hysteroscopic treatment of the symptomatic septate uterus has not only equalled but has surpassed the results obtained with traditional abdominal metroplasties, with over 85% viable pregnancies (12). Furthermore, the patient is spared a laparotomy and hysterotomy, eliminating the potential for pelvic adhesions as well as the associated pain, disability, and expense. Patients treated hysteroscopically need not to wait but one spontaneous menses before attempting conception and do not require a mandatory cesarean section (18–21).

While a larger experience with hysteroscopic division of the uterine septum utilizing hysteroscopic scissors has been accumulated, the results obtained utilizing fiberoptic lasers, such as Argon, KTP-532, and the Nd-YAG, seem to equal the reproductive outcome obtained with hysteroscopic scissors (22–24). The original studies reporting on division of the uterine septum utilizing the resectoscope with a cutting loop eliminated 30% of the patients because of inability to divide all septa, particularly broad ones (13). This restricted treatment may have had to do with the type of electrode used, particularly the 90° resecting loop. The new electrodes are thinner and better designed to reach these areas, and the feasibility rate seems to equal that obtained with hysteroscopic scissors and fiberoptic lasers. Although the choice of instrument depends in part on the familiarity and experience of the operator with various modalities, historically, the use of hysteroscopic scissors for division of the uterine septum has been favored by the majority of physicians performing this type of operation (Tables 8-4, 8-5).

CONCURRENT PROCEDURES

The laparoscope is an excellent adjunct in monitoring the surgical treatment of the symptomatic septate uterus. It allows visualization

TABLE 8-4

Hysteroscopic Division of Uterine Septa (Comparison of Methods)

FEATURE	SCISSORS	RESECTOSCOPE	FIBEROPTIC LASERS
Simplicity	+ +	+	+
Speed	+ + +	+ +	+
Hemostasis	+	+ + +	+ + +
Applicable to all septa	+ +	+	+ +
Evaluation of juxtaposed myometrium	+ + +	+	+
Expense	+	+ +	+ + +
Possible uterine perforation	+	+ +	+ +
Required skill	+ + +	+ + +	+ + +
Fluid overload	+	+ +	+ +

TABLE 8-5

Hysteroscopic Metroplasty

Author	Number Patients	Medium	Technique	IUD*	E/P†	Antibiotics	Pregnancy			
							Term	Premature	Abortion	In Progress
Edstrom (1974)	2	dextran 70, 32%	Rigid biopsy forceps	+	–	–	–	19 wks	–	–
Chervenak and Neuwirth (1981)	2	dextran 70, 32%	Scissors adjacent to hysteroscope	+	+	+	1	–	–	–
Rosenberg et al. (1981)	1	dextran 70, 32%	Flexible scissors	NA§	NA	NA	NA	–	–	–
Daly et al. (1983)	25	dextran 70, 32%	—	–	+	–	7	–	1	2
Perino et al. (1985)	11	CO_2	Flexible, semi-rigid scissors	+	–	–	NA	–	–	–
DeCherney et al. (1986)	72	dextran 70, 32%	Resectoscope	–	–	–	58	–	4	4
Corson and Batzer (1986)	18	dextran 70, 32% CO_2	Resectoscope and rigid scissors	–	–	–	10	1	2	2

Author	N	Distending media	Instrument							
Fayez (1986)	19	dextran 70, 32%	Rigid scissors	Foley catheter	–	+	14	–	–	–
March and Israel (1987)	91	dextran 70, 32%	Flexible scissors	+	+	–	44	4	7	7
Valle (1987)	59	D$_5$W/dextran 70, 32%	Flexible, semi-rigid, rigid scissors	–	+	+	44	2	5	–
Choe and Baggish (1992)	19	dextran 70, 32%	Nd-YAG with bare or sculptured fibers	Foley catheter (3 patients)	+	+	10	1	1	3
Fedele et al. (1993)	102	dextran 40, 10% in normal saline	Semi-rigid scissors (80) Argon Laser (10) Resectoscope (12)	+ (21)	+ (39)	+	45	10	11	NA
Totals	421						233	19	31	18

*IUD = Intrauterine device
†EP = Estrogens/Progesterone
§NA = Nonapplicable

of the external uterine pathology (ruling out a bicornuate uterus), and myometrial thickness (by transillumination) as well as revealing tubal-peritoneal pathology and monitoring the division of the uterine septa in order to decrease the risk of uterine perforation. Sonography has also been used for this purpose, but maintaining the transducer on the same plane with the hysteroscope is cumbersome. Maintaining appropriate uterine planes where the uterine wall and septum can be seen simultaneously is difficult, particularly when the uterus moves as the hysteroscopist proceeds with the division of the septum. Nonetheless, intraoperative sonography will increase the safety of performing these procedures, should laparoscopy be contraindicated. No additional benefit to visualize the pelvic structures can be added by sonography, except in observing enlargement of the ovaries and evaluation of possible ovarian cysts.

Pathology associated with the septate uterus requires the same treatment as that for the lesions alone. Nonetheless, it is advantageous to treat other lesions, such as polyps or myomas, before the uterine septum is divided. This is done in order to allow a more perfect visualization of the symmetry of both uterine cavities. Occasionally, the septum has to be excised first to permit better visualization of the lesions in a unified uterine cavity.

REFERENCES

1. Moore KL. The developing human. Clinically oriented embryology. The urogenital system. 4th ed. Philadelphia: WB Saunders, 1988:246–285.
2. Rock JA, Zacur HA. The clinical management of repeated early pregnancy wastage. Fertil Steril 1983;39:123–140.
3. Carp HJA, Toder V, Mashiach S, Nebel L, Serr DM. Recurrent miscarriage: a review of current concepts, immune mechanisms, and results of treatment. Obstet Gynecol Surv 1990;45:657–669.
4. Buttram VC, Gibbons WE. Müllerian anomalies: a proposed classification (an analysis of 144 cases). Fertil Steril 1979;32:40–46.
5. Valle RF. Clinical management of uterine factors in infertile patients.

In: Speroff L, ed. Seminars in reproductive endocrinology. New York: Georg Thieme Verlag, 1985;3:149–167.

6. Jones AW, Jones GES. Double uterus as an etiologic factor in repeated abortions: indications for surgical repair. Am J Obstet Gynecol 1953;65:325–339.

7. Tompkins P. Comments on the bicornuate uterus and twinning. Surg Clin North Am 1962;42:1049–1062.

8. Daly DC, Walters CA, Soto-Albors CE, Riddick DH. Hysteroscopic metroplasty: surgical technique and obstetric outcome. Fertil Steril 1983;39:623–628.

9. Valle RF, Sciarra JJ. Hysteroscopic treatment of the septate uterus. Obstet Gynecol 1986;676:253–257.

10. Perino A, Mencaglia L, Hamou J, Cittadini E. Hysteroscopy for metroplasty of uterine septa: report of 24 cases. Fertil Steril 1987;48:321–323.

11. Daly DC, Tohan N, Walters C, Riddick DH. Hysteroscopic resection of the uterine septum in the presence of a septate cervix. Fertil Steril 1983;39:560–563.

12. March CM, Israel R. Hysteroscopic management of recurrent abortion caused by septate uterus. Am J Obstet Gynecol 1987;156:834–842.

13. DeCherney AH, Russell JB, Graebe RA, Polan ML. Resectoscopic management of Müllerian fusion defects. Fertil Steril 1986;45:726–728.

14. Rock JA, Murphy AA, Cooper WH. Resectoscopic techniques for the lysis of a class V: complete uterine septum. Fertil Steril 1987;48:495–496.

15. Candiani GB, Vercellini P, Fedele L, et al. Repair of the uterine cavity after hysteroscopic septal incision. Fertil Steril 1990;54:991–994.

16. Candiani GB, Vercellini P, Fidele L, Garsia S, Brioschi D, Villa L. Argon laser versus microscissors for hysteroscopic incision of uterine septa. Am J Obstet Gynecol 1991;164:87–90.

17. Garry R, Hasham F, Kokri MS, Mooney P. The effect of pressure on fluid absorption during endometrial ablation. J Gynecol Surg 1992;8:1–10.

18. Daly DC, Maier D, Soto-Albors C. Hysteroscopic metroplasty: six years experience. Obstet Gynecol 1989;73:201–205.

19. Hysteroscopic metroplasty. In: Siegler AM, Valle RF, Lindemann HJ, Mencaglia L. Therapeutic hysteroscopy. Indications and techniques. St. Louis: CV Mosby, 1990;62–81.

20. Hassiakos DK, Zourlas PA. Transcervical division of the uterine septa. Obstet Gynecol Surv 1990;45:165–173.
21. Fayez JA. Comparison between abdominal and hysteroscopic metroplasty. Obstet Gynecol 1986;68:399–403.
22. Daniell JF, Osher S, Miller W. Hysteroscopic resection of uterine septi with visible light laser energy. Colposc Gynecol Laser Surg 1987;3:217–220.
23. Choe JK, Baggish MS. Hysteroscopic treatment of septate uterus with neodymium–YAG laser. Fertil Steril 1992;57:81–84.
24. Fedele L, Arcaini L, Parazzini F, et al. Reproductive prognosis after hysteroscopic metroplasty in 102 women: lifetable analysis. Fertil Steril 1993;59:768–772.

9

Intrauterine Adhesions

Rafael F. Valle

I ntrauterine adhesions may interfere with both normal reproduction and menstrual patterns. When surgical treatment is undertaken, results are much improved if the corrective surgery is done under direct visualization using a hysteroscope.

ETIOLOGY

Intrauterine adhesions are scars that result from trauma to a recently pregnant uterus. In over 90% of the cases, they are caused by curettage (1–3). Usually, the trauma has occurred because of excessive bleeding requiring curettage 1 to 4 weeks after a delivery of a term or preterm pregnancy or during an abortion. During this vulnerable phase of the endometrium, any trauma may denude or remove the basalis endometrium, causing the uterine walls to adhere to each other and form a permanent bridge, distorting the symmetry of the uterine cavity. In rare circumstances, conditions such as abdominal metroplasties or myomectomies may cause intrauterine adhesions, but these adhesions are usually due to misplaced sutures rather than the true coaptation of denuded areas of myometrium that occurs following postpartum or postabortal curettage (3).

The type and consistency of these adhesions vary: some are focal, some extensive, some mild, and some thickened and dense, with extensive fibromuscular or connective tissue components. The extent and type of uterine cavity occlusion correlate well with the extent of trauma during the vulnerable phase of the endometrium following a recent pregnancy. Some adhesions are focal, others completely occlude the uterine cavity. Consistency usually follows the longevity and duration of these adhesions, the older ones being thickened and dense and formed by connective tissue (4–7).

Reproductive outcome seems to correlate well with the type of adhesions and the extent of uterine cavity occlusion. Therefore, it is useful to have a way of classifying these adhesions as filmy and composed endometrial tissue, fibromuscular, or composed of connective tissue. The degree of uterine cavity occlusion is also important. Attempts to classify intrauterine adhesions by hysterosalpingography give a good appraisal of the extent of uterine cavity occlusion, but it is impossible to determine by hysterosalpingography the type of adhesions that are present. When using hysteroscopy alone, it is difficult to assess the extent of uterine cavity occlusion by visualization because the axis to the hysteroscopist is from the cervix to the fundus and not perpendicular to the uterine body as hysterography is, outlining the uterine cavity from a different axis. For this reason, the combination of hysterosalpingography and hysteroscopy has been used most commonly to assess not only the extent of uterine cavity occlusion, but also the type of adhesions found by hysteroscopy at the time of treatment. Valle and Sciarra (3) utilized a three-stage classification of the extent and severity of intrauterine adhesions (mild, moderate, and severe) based on the degree of involvement shown on hysterosalpingography and the extent and type of adhesions found on hysteroscopy. Three stages of intrauterine adhesions are defined: *Mild adhesions*—filmy adhesions composed of basalis endometrial tissue producing partial or complete uterine cavity occlusion; *moderate adhesions*—fibromuscular adhesions, characteristically thick, still covered with endometrium that may bleed upon division, which partially or totally occlude the uterine cavity; and *severe adhesions*—composed of connective tissue only, lacking any endometrial lining, and not likely to bleed upon division. These adhesions may partially or totally occlude the uterine cavity (3).

Recently, the American Fertility Society has proposed a classification of intrauterine adhesions based on the findings at hysterosalpingography and hysteroscopy and their correlation with menstrual patterns (8). Using a uniform classification for intrauterine adhesions greatly enhances our ability to report, evaluate, and compare results of different treatments of intrauterine adhesions, particularly when utilizing these modalities by the hysteroscopic approach.

INDICATIONS FOR TREATMENT

Intrauterine adhesions frequently result in menstrual abnormalities, such as hypomenorrhea or even amenorrhea, depending upon the extent of uterine cavity occlusion. Patients with long-standing intrauterine adhesions may also develop dysmenorrhea. Over 75% of women with moderate or severe adhesions will have either amenorrhea or hypomenorrhea. Patients with significant uterine cavity occlusion secondary to intrauterine adhesions experience menstrual abnormalities, particularly amenorrhea (37%) and hypomenorrhea (31%). Patients with minimal or focal intrauterine adhesions may not demonstrate obvious menstrual abnormalities and may continue to have normal menses (9).

Patients may also exhibit problems in reproduction, particularly pregnancy wastage, should the adhesions not totally occlude the uterine cavity. When total amenorrhea and total uterine cavity occlusion exist, the patient will generally be infertile. Other problems associated with intrauterine adhesions are premature labor, fetal demise, and ectopic pregnancy. When pregnancy is carried to term, placental insertion abnormalities, such as placenta accreta, percreta, or increta may occur. Schenker and Margalioth (9) evaluated 292 patients who did not receive treatment for intrauterine adhesions. Of these, 133 women conceived (45.5%), and of these, only 50 (30%) achieved a term pregnancy; 38 (23%) had preterm labor, and 66 patients had a spontaneous abortion (40%). In 21 patients (13%), placenta previa, ectopic pregnancy, and abnormal placental insertions, such as placenta accreta, were diagnosed.

The most important clue to the diagnosis of intrauterine adhesions is a history of trauma to the endometrial cavity, particularly following delivery or abortion. Secondary to that is a history of amenorrhea or hypomenorrhea. Because intrauterine adhesions are not related to hormonal events, an intact hypothalamic-pituitary-ovarian axis should result in a biphasic basal body temperature chart demonstrating ovulation; failure to withdraw from a progesterone challenge test in a patient who is amenorrheic will strengthen the diagnosis. Uterine sounding has been used to ascertain obstruction of the internal cervical os, but this test should be abandoned because of an increased danger of uterine perforation as well as inaccuracy of diagnosis. The most useful screening test for intrauterine adhesions is a hysterosalpingogram. It provides evaluation of the internal cervical os and uterine cavity, delineation of the adhesions, and information about the condition of the rest of the uterine cavity if adhesions do not completely occlude this area. About 1.5% of hysterosalpingograms performed for infertility evaluation demonstrate intrauterine adhesions (10). When hysterosalpingograms are performed for repeated abortions, about 5% demonstrate intrauterine adhesions (9). A history compatible with intrauterine adhesions will increase the yield of hysterosalpingography for intrauterine adhesions in about 39% of patients (11). These adhesions are star-like, stellate irregular shaped, filling defects, with ragged contours and variable locations in the uterine cavity. They are most commonly found in the central corporeal cavity and less frequently at the uterotubal cones and lower uterine segment.

Despite the usefulness of hysterosalpingography as a screening method for patients suspected of having intrauterine adhesions, the final diagnosis is determined only by direct visualization with hysteroscopy because about 30% of abnormal hysterosalpingograms may be excluded by hysteroscopy (12). The diagnosis can be confirmed by visualization, and the appropriate treatment can be provided once the adhesions are observed endoscopically.

Hysterosalpingography is useful in determining the extent of uterine cavity occlusion, but it cannot provide an appraisal of the consistency and type of intrauterine adhesions. For this reason, hysteroscopy becomes a useful adjunct to hysterosalpingography by confirming the extent and type of intrauterine adhesions.

Other techniques, such as ultrasonography and magnetic resonance imaging (MRI), have been used to make this diagnosis, but their accuracy is not well determined, and not enough experience exists with these techniques to supplant the hysterosalpingogram and hysteroscopy (13,14). Furthermore, the cost may be prohibitive.

METHODS OF TREATMENT

Treatment of intrauterine adhesions is surgical, consisting of removing those adhesions by division. In the past, blind methods of division were used with curettes, probes or dilators, or hysterotomy-assisted division of these adhesions under direct vision, but these techniques have failed to produce acceptable results and have been largely abandoned. Introduction of modern hysteroscopy has permitted transcervical division of adhesions under visual guidance; hysteroscopic methods have used mechanical means, such as hysteroscopic scissors, the resectoscope, and fiberoptic lasers.

Treatment of intrauterine adhesions with hysteroscopic scissors is the most common method employed. Because intrauterine adhesions, in general, are avascular and divided (not removed), the treatment has been similar to that for division of a uterine septum. The adhesions are divided centrally, allowing the uterine cavity to expand upon division of the adhesions. This is performed utilizing flexible, semi-rigid and, occasionally, rigid or optical scissors. The most commonly used method is the semi-rigid hysteroscopic scissors because of the increased facility manipulating the scissors, selectively dividing these adhesions when they retract upon cutting. Occasionally, thick connective tissue adhesions are present that form very thick stumps and benefit not only from division but also from removal. To achieve this effect, a biopsy forceps sometimes becomes most useful when lateral thick adhesions are present, and the technique involves not only division of the adhesions but also removal. It is important to use a sharp biospy forceps to selectively sculpture the uterine cavity to achieve a uniform symmetry. This technique is also useful at the uterotubal cones, particularly at the junction of the tubal openings and the uterus (Figures 9-1 to 9-4).

While the semi-rigid and flexible scissors are most useful for the division of adhesions by hysteroscopy, the rigid optical scissors are less helpful in this endeavor. Because of the thick, sturdy configuration of these adhesions, when the uterine wall is thin and sclerotic, there is greater chance of uterine perforation, particularly because a panoramic view is impaired. Targeted dissection, which is easily obtained with the flexible and semi-rigid scissors, is hampered and difficult with optical scissors.

Fluids with electrolytes should be used when dividing these adhesions because of increased chances of intravasation and because the adhesions are cut close to the myometrial tissue, and the extensive area of denudation may predispose to fluid intravasation. Normal saline, dextrose 5% in half normal saline, and Ringer's lactate

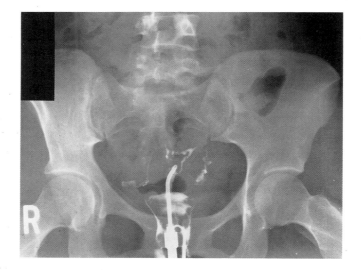

FIGURE 9-1

Hysterosalpingogram shows extensive uterine cavity occlusion by adhesions.

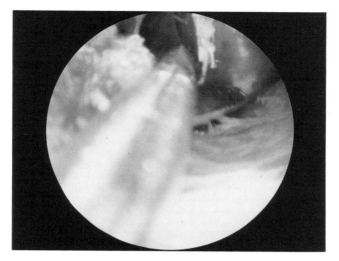

FIGURE 9-2

Hysteroscopic division of extensive intrauterine adhesions using semi-rigid scissors.

A B

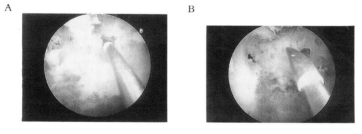

FIGURE 9-3

Hysteroscopic division of extensive fundal intrauterine adhesions: (a) initial division of adhesions; (b) right uterotubal cone is visible.

are most appropriate. Care must be taken to measure the amount of fluid used and the amount recovered when using the hysteroscope, particularly if the instrument has inflow and outflow, permitting an estimate of the amount of fluid that has been intravasated. In the absence of a continuous flow system, care must be taken to measure the total inflow of fluids and ascertain that the intrauterine pressure does not exceed the mean arterial pressure of about 100 mmHg.

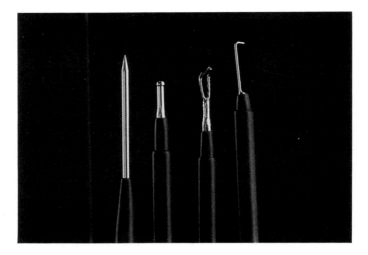

FIGURE 9-4

Electrodes for use through hysteroscopic operating channel (6.0 French, 2 mm). Left to right: point tip, ball tip, loop tip, hook tip (courtesy of Cook Ob/Gyn).

These procedures must be expedited to avoid excessive intravasation of fluid.

Depending upon the extent of uterine cavity occlusion, division is done under visual control by cutting the adhesions in the middle to avoid uterine damage at the level of the uterine wall. When there is total uterine cavity occlusion, selective dissection of adhesions begins at the internal cervical os until a neocavity is created and then the dissection progresses until the uterotubal cones are free. When extensive adhesions are present, the hysteroscopist should be alert to perforation. Concomitant laparoscopy should be considered in all cases. Upon completion of the procedure, indigo carmine is injected transcervically to test for tubal patency.

The procedure is performed by systematically dividing the adhesions and cutting as much as feasible, particularly when there is total uterine cavity occlusion (3,15).

The advantages of using hysteroscopic scissors for the division of intrauterine adhesions are those of mechanical methods. Mechanical tools provide excellent landmarks when dividing these adhesions, particularly when approaching the juxtaposed myometrium. Bleeding may be observed at the myometrium, and this warns the hysteroscopist to stop the dissection so as to avoid perforation. No scattering of energies is produced to damage the small areas of healthy endometrium, which are the reservoir for future reepithelialization. This is an important consideration because no extensive healthy endometrium can be found when extensive intrauterine adhesions are present. The disadvantages are that it may sometimes be difficult to manipulate semirigid instrumentation, particularly to the lateral walls of the uterine cavity. Scissors do not provide the sharpness or mechanism to cut these adhesions, as the scissors do not close well distally and need to be readjusted and sharpened frequently.

Treatment of intrauterine adhesions utilizing the resectoscope is an alternative to mechanical tools. The resectoscope can be used to divide intrauterine adhesions either with a resecting loop, a loop bent forward, or with specifically designed electrodes that can be directly applied to the adhesions dividing them easily. These are in the form of knives or wires that must be specifically and selectively directed to the adhesions, particularly those in the lateral portion of the uterus or at the uterotubal cones. When utilizing the resectoscope, fluids without electrolytes must be used, e.g., dextrose 5% in water, glycine 1.5%, or sorbitol 3.5%, which provide excellent visualization and are useful distending media. When dividing these adhesions, the resectoscopic loop may not be the appropriate electrode to use because it is designed to resect rather than to selectively divide centrally the adhesions. When the resectoscopic loop has been used, several complications occur, particularly due to future sacculations of the uterus, dehiscences, and perforations. Ascertaining where the adhesions finish and when the normal myometrium begins is difficult, and the resections may be so deep that a portion of the myometrium must be shaved during division of the uterine septum. Electrodes, such as the knife types or wire types that can selectively be directed to the adhesions and divide them systematically, have been specifically designed for this purpose. Nonetheless, concern remains about scattering the energy and damaging the peripheral healthy endometrium. With the use of specific electrodes, this effect may be somewhat decreased. It is important to monitor the operation with concomitant laparoscopy because the landmarks of junction between adhesions and myometrium may be lost, and the coagulating effect this energy may produce in the myometrium may obscure a view of small vessels that, when bleeding, warn the hysteroscopist to stop further dissection.

Use of the resectoscope has several advantages. Bleeding is decreased during dissection because of the electrical coagulating effect. The resectoscopic continuous flow system allows estimation of the deficit of fluid, thus decreasing the chances of fluid overload.

There are also disadvantages. Monopolar energy must be used. Only fluids devoid of electrolytes can be used. Additionally, electrosurgical damage of peripheral endometrium and the loss of landmarks while coagulating close to the myometrium, resulting in inadvertent invasion of this area may occur. Finally, electrical damage to surrounding organs with or without perforation is a risk (16).

Treatment of intrauterine adhesions with fiberoptic lasers, such as the Nd-YAG, Argon, and KTP/532, can also be used to divide intrauterine adhesions. However, their application has been somewhat limited. The Nd-YAG laser with sculptured or extruded fibers can be a useful tool to selectively divide intrauterine adhesions, particularly those that are lateral and fundal (15). Care must be taken to use these fibers by contact and selectively be aware of the overall symmetry of the uterine cavity because the coagulating power of the laser may cause a similar effect to electrosurgery; that is, coagulation and cutting, and the landmarks of the juxtaposed myometrium may be lost while performing division of the adhesions. Small arteries that cross the myometrium may not bleed, so dissection may proceed further than necessary. The hysteroscopic manipulation of the fiberoptic lasers is very easy and is facilitated with the use of foroblique telescopes. The Argon and KTP-532 utilize the sharpest fibers to cut rather than to coagulate (17).

Because lasers are not conductive, fluids with electrolytes should be used. Normal saline, dextrose 5% in half normal saline, or Ringer's lactate provide excellent visualization and contain sodium if excessive fluids are absorbed. The utilization of these electrolyte-containing fluids will not prevent pulmonary edema but will decrease the risk of hyponatremia; therefore, more fluid may be used than when using fluids without electrolytes. Ideally, a hysteroscope with a continuous flow system should be used—or one with true inflow and outflow—to collect the injected fluid and have a perfect account of the deficit or nonrecovered fluid.

Use of the laser is attractive and has the benefit of easy manipulation, but requires more time than use of mechanical tools, such as hysteroscopic scissors. It is important, therefore, when utilizing this type of energy to expedite the procedure as much as possible, so as to avoid excessive fluid from being intravasated.

INTRA- AND POSTGENERATIVE MANAGEMENT

The principal goal of therapy is to remove the adhesions surgically. Because most of these patients have a sclerotic or destroyed endometrium, they need other adjunctive therapy to promote re-epithelialization and a mechanical separation of the uterine walls to prevent the reformation of adhesions. These adjuncts are intrauterine splints, prophylactic antibiotics, estrogens, and progesterone, to promote re-epithelialization.

Prophylactic antibiotics are used routinely in these patients in view of a traumatized endometrium and the extensive manipulation these patients usually require. The antibiotics used are in the form of cephalosporins, Kefzol 1 mg IV piggyback one half hour before the procedure, to be followed with Keflex 500 mg q.i.d. PO for a week. Additionally, in those patients with extensive intrauterine adhesions, an indwelling number 8 pediatic Foley catheter is inserted and 3 to 3½ mL of a solution instilled. It is left in place for a week to prevent reformation of adhesions. Adjunctive hormonal therapy consists of natural estrogens in the form of Premarin 2.5 mg b.i.d. for 30 or 40 days, depending on the extent of uterine cavity occlusion and the type of adhesions found. The more extensive and old the adhesions are, the more prolonged the hormonal treatment needed. In the last 10 days of this artificial cycle, medroxyprogesterone acetate (Provera) 10 mg a day are given PO for 10 days. Upon completion of the hormonal treatment, and once withdrawal bleeding has ceased, a hysterosalpingogram is performed to assess the results of the operation and decide upon further therapy or initiation of attempts to conception. Those patients with filmy, focal adhesions may not require hysterosalpingography but an office hysteroscopy to assess uterine cavity symmetry (3,18).

RESULTS

The results of hysteroscopic treatment of intrauterine adhesions have correlated well with the extent of uterine cavity occlusion and the type of adhesions present. Normal menstruation is restored in over 90% of the patients (3,18). The reproductive outcome correlates well with the type of adhesions and the extent of uterine cavity occlusion. Of 187 patients treated hysteroscopically by Valle and Sciarra (3), removal of mild, filmy adhesions in 43 cases gave the best result, with 35 (81%) term pregnancies; in 97 moderate cases of fibromuscular adhesions, 64 (66%) term pregnancies occurred, and in 47 severe cases of connective tissue adhesions, 15 (32%) term pregnancies occurred. Overall restoration of menses occurred in 90% of the patients, and the overall term pregnancy rate was 79.7%. These results demonstrate a much better reproductive outcome than was previously obtained with blind methods of therapy (Table 9-1).

Results following treatment of intrauterine adhesions utilizing the resectoscope have been similar; nonetheless, the reported postoperative complications may be serious and should be kept in mind when utilizing this type of instrument. A few series report lysis of adhesions with fiberoptic lasers, but when the lasers are used appropriately, results should not vary much from those reported with electrosurgery (16,19).

TABLE 9-1

Hysteroscopic Lysis of Intrauterine Adhesions

Author	No. Patients	Results			NL§ Menses (%)	Reproductive Outcome	
		IUD*	E/P†	Antibiotics		Pregnant (%)	Term (%)
Edstrom (1974)	9	+	–	–	2	1	1
March et al. (1981)	38	+	+	+	38 (100)	38 (100)	34 (79.1)
Neuwirth et al. (1982)	27	+	+	+	20 (74)	14 (51.8)	13 (48.1)
Sanfilippo et al. (1982)	26	+	+	–	26 (100)	6 (100)	3 (50)
Siegler and Kontopoulos (1981)	25	Foley catheter	+	–	13 (52)	11 (44)	6 (24)
Hamou et al. (1983)	69	+	+	–	59 (85.5)	20 (51.3)	15 (38.4)
Sugimoto et al. (1984)	258	+	+	–	180 (69.7)	107 (41.4)	64 (24.8)
Wamsteker (1984)	36	+	+	+	34 (94.4)	17 (62.9)	12 (44.4)
Friedman et al. (1986)	30	–	+	–	27 (90)	24 (80)	23 (76.6)
Valle and Sciarra (1987)	187	+	+	+	167 (89.3)	143 (76.4)	114 (60.9)
Zuanchong and Yulian (1986)	70	Foley catheter	+	+	64 (84.3)	30 (85.7)	17 (48.5)
Totals	775				630 (87.2)	411 (60.3)	302 (44.3)

*IUD = Intrauterine device
†E/P = Estrogens/Progesterone
§NL = Normal

SUMMARY

Hysteroscopic surgery has been greatly facilitated and enhanced by the use of the gynecologic resectoscope. No single technique, used exclusively, can accomplish all tasks. Used in combination with other available techniques for hysteroscopic surgery, however, the gynecologic resectoscope enhances our ability to treat different conditions that required major surgery in the past. The treatment of the symptomatic septate uterus, as well as the treatment of intrauterine adhesions, can be accomplished by three different techniques: scissors, resectoscope, and fiberoptic lasers. All have advantages and disadvantages and must be used with knowledge of each particular technology and its drawbacks. Each technique should be tailored not only to the anatomy, embryology, and etiology of each process but also to the experience and knowledge of the operator. The operator should select the appropriate method and technique for each patient. The goals of therapy should be a successful pregnancy for those patients with impaired reproduction, keeping in mind the safety of the patient, with the least morbidity possible, the absence of complications, the overall effectiveness, and diminution of unnecessary cost. Versatility plays a significant role in the selection of therapeutic alternatives the surgeon has to intelligently select the best method for each individual patient.

REFERENCES

1. Asherman JG. Amenorrhea traumatica (atretica). J Obset Gynaecol Br Emp 1948;55:23–30.
2. Asherman JG. Traumatic intrauterine adhesions. J Obstet Gynaecol Br Emp 1950;57:892–896.
3. Valle RF, Sciarra JJ. Intrauterine adhesions: hysteroscopic diagnosis, classification, treatment, and reproductive outcome. Am J Obstet Gynecol 1988;158:1459–1470.
4. Foix A, Bruno RO, Davidson T, Lema B: The pathology of postcurettage intrauterine adhesions. Am J Obstet Gynecol 1966;96:1027–1033.

5. Siegler AM, Kontopoulos VG. Lysis of intrauterine adhesions under hysteroscopic control: a report of 25 operations. J Reprod Med 1981; 26:372–374.

6. March CM, Israel R, March AD. Hysteroscopic management of intra-uterine adhesions. Am J Obstet Gynecol 1978;130:653.

7. Siegler AM, Valle RF. Therapeutic hysteroscopic procedures. Fertil Steril 1988;50:685–701.

8. The American Fertility Society. Classifications of adnexal adhesions, distal tubal occlusion, tubal occlusion secondary to tubal ligation, tubal pregnancies, Müllerian anomalies, and intrauterine adhesions. Fertil Steril 1988;49:944–955.

9. Schenker JG, Margalioth EJ. Intrauterine adhesions: an updated appraisal. Fertil Steril 1982;37:593–610.

10. Dmowski WP, Greenblatt RB. Asherman's syndrome and risk of placenta accreta. Obstet Gynecol 1969;34:288–299.

11. Klein SM, Garcia CR. Asherman's syndrome: a critique and current review. Fertil Steril 1973;24:722–735.

12. Valle RF, Sciarra JJ. Current status of hysteroscopy in gynecologic practice. Fertil Steril 1979;32:619–632.

13. Confino E, Friberg J, Giglia RV, Gleicher N. Sonographic imaging of intrauterine adhesions. Obstet Gynecol 1985;66:596–598.

14. Vartiainen J, Kajanoja P, Ylostalo PR. Ultrasonography in extended placental retention and intrauterine adhesions: a case report. Eur J Obstet Gynecol Reprod Biol 1989;30:89–93.

15. Neuwirth RS, Hussein AR, Schiffman BM, Amin HK. Hysteroscopic resection of intrauterine scars using a new technique. Obstet Gynecol 1982;60:111–113.

16. Friedman A, Defazio J, DeCherney AH. Severe obstetric complications following hysteroscopic lysis of adhesions. Obstet Gynecol 1986;67:864–867.

17. Newton JR, Mackenzie WE, Emens MJ, Jordan JA. Division of uterine adhesions (Asherman's syndrome) with the Nd-YAG laser. Br J Obstet Gynaecol 1989;96:102–104.

18. March CM, Israel R. Gestational outcome following hysteroscopic lysis of adhesions. Fertil Steril 1981;36:455.

19. Intrauterine adhesions. In: Siegler AM, Valle RF, Lindemann HJ, Mencaglia L. Therapeutic hysteroscopy. Indications and techniques. St. Louis: CV Mosby, 1990:82–105.

10

Removing Intrauterine Lesions: Myomectomy and Polypectomy

Franklin D. Loffer

P rior to hysteroscopy, many intrauterine polyps and myoma went undiagnosed until the patient came to hysterectomy. Blind procedures, such as endometrial biopsies and dilatation and curettage, do not detect the majority of intrauterine growths (1,2). Imaging procedures are more helpful. Unfortunately, the false-positive rate may be high, and lesions identified at a hysterogram are proven hysteroscopically or by hysterectomy in only 43% to 69% of cases (3,4,5). Newer diagnostic techniques, such as ultrasound, are better tools than the hystograms for determining the nature of an intrauterine lesion (6,7,8). The expense of MRIs precludes their use for this purpose. None of the imaging techniques provide tissue for pathological diagnosis.

Hysteroscopy is an excellent method for not only identifying intrauterine lesions but also for removing them. The first suggestion that a transcervical approach using a resection loop could be used was in 1957 (9). Although the instrument was not clearly described, specific reference was made that it was not a urological resectoscope. The first reported gynecological use of a resection loop was in 1978, when a urological resectoscope was used (10). Subsequent to that time, other reports have been published (11–32).

ANATOMY

It is necessary to understand the anatomy of the intrauterine lesions that will be found and treated in order to select what cases are appropriate for hysteroscopic management and in what manner the resectoscope will be used. Intrauterine growths are defined as being either pedunculated or sessile. This distinction is based on their attachment to the uterine wall. A *pedunculated structure* is attached by a stalk or pedicle. A *sessile structure* is one whose attachment is by a broad base.

A polypoid structure may be a leiomyoma, an adenomyoma, or an endometrial polyp. The differentiation between pedunculated and sessile leiomyoma is a matter of the size of the stalk, since leiomyoma are intimately related to myometrium and demarcated by a false or pseudocapsule. This capsule is less well demonstrated in those leiomyomas that are pedunculated. Pedunculated adenomyomas of the uterus are a mixture of normal endometrium and uterine musculature, which contain endometrial glands without any surrounding endometrial stroma. Like leiomyomas, they also may be sessile. They frequently occur in young patients and may be the basis of infertility. Endometrial polyps originate from the middle or basal third of the endometrium and may or may not be covered by the functioning endometrium.

Sessile leiomyomas and adenomyomas lie partially embedded in the myometrium. The amount embedded can be estimated by the angle the leiomyoma makes with the endometrium at its attachment to the uterine wall. A simple grading scale has been proposed (33). Those leiomyomas that lie primarily or completely within the uterine wall are intramural and not approachable by hysteroscopic techniques. Subserosal leiomyomas, which lie beyond the uterine cavity on the abdominal side of the uterus, are also not suitable for hysteroscopic management.

Although very uncommon, both endometrial polyps and leiomyomas may show malignant changes. The author found one case in his first 101 patients. The risk of malignancy would appear to be as high as 1% (34) to 1.6% (22). There are no specific characteristics to identify malignancy prior to tissue being sent for pathological review.

Sessile and pedunculated lesions can arise from anywhere in the uterine cavity. On occasion, pedunculated lesions in the lower uterine segment may prolapse through the cervix and be visible on vaginal examination.

Hysteroscopists often discuss the maximum size of a myoma that can be successfully resected. It is the author's opinion that the size of the submucous myoma is relatively self-limiting. If it is primarily intramural, it can grow to any size since it will enlarge the uterus and further distort the uterine cavity. Intramural myomas are not managed by hysteroscopy. However, when the myoma is primarily intrauterine, it can grow until it reaches a size of 4 to 6 cm. At that time, it will be prolapsed through the cervical canal (Figure 10-1). Although myomas larger than 4 to 6 cm may be identified by ultrasound to be projecting into the cavity, they probably are primarily intramural and, therefore, not good candidates for hysteroscopic resection.

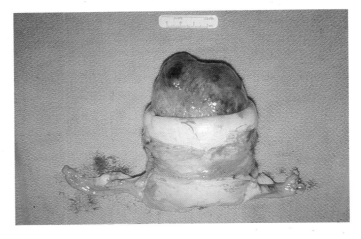

FIGURE 10-1

The size of submucous myomas is probably self-limiting. This fibroid measuring approximately 6 cm could no longer be contained in the uterine cavity.

INDICATIONS FOR
HYSTEROSCOPIC SURGERY

Patients with intrauterine lesions will generally present with either abnormal bleeding, pregnancy wastage/infertility, or both. Occasionally, a pelvic ultrasound performed for pelvic pain or to evaluate the adnexa or the size of uterine leiomyoma may identify an as yet asymptomatic intrauterine lesion.

The usual history given by premenopausal patients who present with abnormal bleeding is progressively heavier periods associated with increasing pre- and postmenstrual spotting and length of flow. Some of the heaviest menstrual bleeding patients experience is related to submucous leiomyoma. Postmenopausal patients may present with postmenopausal bleeding or excessively heavy withdrawal bleeding from hormonal replacement therapy.

The initial evaluation of premenopausal patients presenting with significant menorrhagia or menometrorrhagia is usually not surgical. If the bleeding is of recent onset and not severe, observation may be indicated. If the bleeding continues, it should be determined if medical therapy can control the problem. When the bleeding is related to anovulation, endocrine causes should be ruled out. If no underlying correctable problem is identified, cyclic progesterone or oral contraceptives can be given to regulate and decrease the menstrual flow. A diagnostic hysteroscopy is indicated when the menorrhagia or menometrorrhagia fails conservative treatment, is persistent, severe, or occurs in a postmenopausal patient. This hysteroscopic evaluation can usually be done in an office setting.

Some patients who want hysteroscopic surgical management of their bleeding problems and in whom infertility is not a concern may choose not to have an office hysteroscopy. They can first be evaluated by hysteroscopy in an outpatient facility prior to the expected definitive surgery. This alternative is feasible since the cause of the bleeding is usually from a submucous leiomyoma or a normal appearing endometrial cavity, and the menorrhagia can usually be managed at the time of the initial diagnosis. If a lesion is present, it can be removed. If no lesion is present, an endometrial ablation can be done. It is important that patients who choose this route understand there may be findings that preclude any hysteroscopic management. This risk can be minimized. A preoperative endometrial biopsy will determine ovulation and rule out premalignant changes. Sounding of the uterus can determine size of the cavity and, if large, suggests a submucous fibroid. An ultrasound will also provide further information.

In patients whose only complaint is infertility or pregnancy wastage, screening hysteroscopy has little value (4). The initial evaluation should generally be a hystosalpingogram. If a filling defect is found, it can then be evaluated and managed hysteroscopically. Most patients with pregnancy wastage or infertility secondary to an intrauterine lesion will have associated menorrhagia, and clinical suspicion will be raised that an intrauterine lesion may exist.

SURGICAL METHODS

Intrauterine lesions have been removed by a variety of methods. Enucleation of lesions with scissors has been described (35). The Nd–YAG laser has been successfully used with sapphire tips (Surgical Laser Technology Corporation, Malvern, PA) (Loffer FD, unpublished observations) and bare fibers (36–38). The energy from the Nd–YAG laser can be used to transect the base of polypoid lesions, transect sessile lesions into small pieces, or necrose larger lesions. Polyp snares may also be used in both pedunculated and sessile lesions (39). Hysteroscopic evaluation of the uterine cavity to identify the location of the lesions followed by wide dilatation with laminaria will also allow a ring forcep to be placed in the uterine cavity and the lesion evulsed from the uterine cavity (40).

However, it is the resectoscope that is most ideally designed to remove intrauterine lesions. Although the resectoscope requires more dilatation than scissors, snares, or the Nd–YAG laser, it is generally more versatile. It requires less cervical dilation and is, therefore, probably less potentially damaging to the cervix than the evulsion technique. It is suitable for all operable lesions and, when appropriate waveform and power settings are used, will limit the area of surrounding tissue destruction (see Chapter 4). The continuous flow resectoscope should always allow adequate visualization, even when patients are bleeding heavily. Hemostasis from the transected area is easily obtained, and the chips can be sent to pathology for histological review. Because of these features, most hysteroscopists are now using the resectoscope for the removal of uterine leiomyomas and endometrial polyps.

TECHNIQUES OF USING THE RESECTOSCOPE

Patient preparation prior to surgery does not need to be extensive. A few authors use laminaria to soften and dilate the cervix prior to the procedure (24,26). Prophylactic antibiotics are often used (12,13,16, 18,22,26,30,31) but many others do not use them and have not reported increased infections (21,23–25,28). However, antibiotics may be of advantage in patients with a past history of pelvic inflammatory disease (41). When a very large fibroid is to be resected, an effort can be made to reduce its size with the use of leuprolide acetate (TAP Pharmaceutical) (see Chapter 7).

The uterine cavity is normally distended with a low viscosity nonelectrolyte-containing fluid, such as sorbitol, glycine, or mannitol. A diluted dextran 70 solution or dextrose and water can also be used. Undiluted dextran 70 and CO_2 are not suited for use with the continuous flow resectoscope. Water should not used as intravasation will cause intravascular hemolysis.

Resectoscopic equipment has been described in detail elsewhere (see Chapter 2). The usual telescope used has a foroblique lens with an angle of view ranging between 12° and 30°. A zero degree endoscope can also be used (18). It is the author's preference to use a 30° telescope. Although this makes observation of the fully extended electrode more difficult, it does make it easier to look behind polyps and fibroids and to see where they lie in the uterine cavity.

The usual electrode used is a 90° loop. The electrode is advanced beyond the end of the telescope by moving the thumb ring forward. When fully extended, it may start to leave the field of view. When pressure on the thumb ring is relaxed, the built-in tension of the instrument will cause the loop to traverse back towards the end of the telescope and be withdrawn into the insulated end of the resectoscope. In order to resect the largest amount of tissue possible at any given time, the loop electrode will have to be placed behind the material to be cut. It is often troubling to the novice hysteroscopist that the loop is then hidden by the tissue to be resected. It must be remembered that the loop is usually electrically activated only when being brought towards the end of the telescope. Therefore, only the tissue lying between the outstretched loop and the end of the telescope will be transected (Figure 10-2). Occasionally, in order to undercut a piece of tissue, the electronically activated loop may be advanced for a *short* distance under *direct* vision.

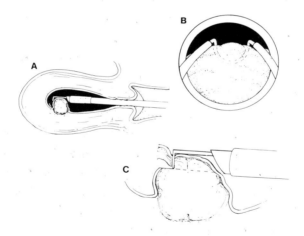

FIGURE 10-2

Placement of the loop electrode to maximize the size of the chip. (a) In order for the largest possible chip to be obtained, it is necessary to place the loop behind the lesion to be transected. (b) Although the loop is out of sight, the depth is limited by the supporting arms of the electrode. (c) The only tissue that will be cut is that which lies between the end of the resectoscope and the electrode.

If there is any question as to where the loop lies in relationship to other structures, such as the tubal ostia, it is possible, using a 30° telescope, to advance the loop only slightly beyond the end of the telescope and to place it under direct vision. Then, while advancing, the loop is advanced at the same speed that the resectoscope is withdrawn. This results in the loop staying in the same position as initially placed but positioned, fully extended from the end of the resectoscope. This maneuver allows a full cut to be obtained (Figure 10-3).

In the above descriptions while cutting chips, the resectoscope does not move in relationship to the uterine cavity—only the electrode is moved. At times, when a lesion is particularly large, it is advantageous to start the resection as described above, and when the loop is approximately halfway towards the end of the telescope, the whole resectoscope can be withdrawn a short distance before the electrode is allowed to close into the end of the instruments (Figure 10-4).

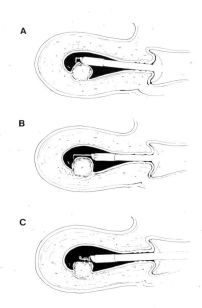

FIGURE 10-3

Placing the electrode under direct vision. (a) The electrode is placed under direct vision; (b) the resectoscope is withdrawn at the same speed the electrode is advanced. This results in the loop being fully extended without altering the placement of the electrode. (c) Resection can now be done.

Removing Intrauterine Lesions: Myomectomy and Polypectomy   175

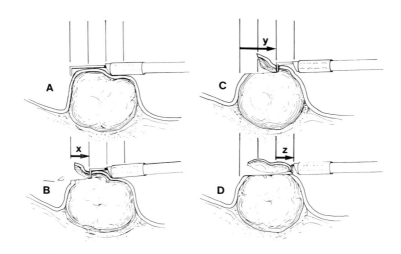

FIGURE 10-4

Increasing the length of chips removed by movement of both the electrode and the resectoscope. (a) The loop is placed fully extended (see illustration 10-2 a, b); (b) the loop is partially closed resecting a portion (x) of the chip; (c) the resectoscope is then withdrawn without further closing of the loop thus enlarging the length of the chip to y; (d) finally, the loop is closed into the resectoscope completing the formation of a long chip by resecting to z.

As tissue is cut, it frequently will pull up against the end of the telescope and momentarily obstruct view. When this occurs, visualization can be achieved by advancing the electrode without any electrical current being applied. Another troublesome problem is that tissue will frequently stick to the electrode. When this occurs, it may fall free when the loop is repositioned for the next resection. If it does not, it will separate as soon as the next resection is begun.

Generally, power settings of 100 to 110 watts of a continuous (cut) current provides a good cutting effect. Since the electrode is literally cutting through tissue on a bed of sparks, the operator should feel little resistance as the loop comes back towards the resectoscope (see Chapter 4). In order to facilitate this arcing, the foot pedal of the generator should be keyed just prior to the electrode making contact with the tissue to be resected. If the operator feels the electrode is dragging as it passes through the tissue, either the power setting is too low or the electrode is being drawn too quickly through the tissue. A blend waveform is not necessary since bleeding from the transected surfaces is seldom a problem. Occasionally, however, a smaller arterial bleeder will be visualized as a small geyser of blood. The loop can be placed against this and a short burst of 40 W of a modulated (coagulating) current will be sufficient to stop the bleeding.

Bubbles and other small debris can be a problem, especially when working on the anterior surface of the uterine cavity. It is the continuous flow design of the gynecological resectoscope that allows the cavity to be quickly cleaned by a rapid turnover of the distending media.

It is the author's preference to distend the uterus with low viscosity media using gravity feed. Mechanical pumps may be used, but they do not provide additional safety. The bag of distending media is raised approximately one meter over the level of the patient. A wide bore Y-shaped urological tubing must be used. This generates a pressure of approximately 75 mmHg with an adequate flow rate and allows for changing of new bags without disruption of flow of distending media. The outflow part of the resectoscope is connected to wall suction. This not only allows for the measurement of the amount of fluids removed from the uterus but facilitates the cleansing of the cavity. The outflow is generally kept partially closed to reduce the amount of fluid used. When necessary to rapidly clear the cavity of bloody bubbles or debris, it can temporarily be opened fully.

When sessile lesions are at the top of the uterine fundus, it may be difficult to shave them down with a 90° electrode. One hundred and eighty degree electrodes are available. No thumb action is required with a 180° electrode except to advance the tip beyond the end of the telescope in order to provide adequate visualization. Movement of the scope from one side to the other will then allow the electrode to shave the fundal fibroid to the level of the uterine cavity.

When a polypoid structure is being removed, it is possible to transect the base by dropping the 90° electrode into the stalk. It may be necessary to do this in more than one side of the stalk. Frequently, part of the stalk remains after the body of the polyp is removed. It can then be shaved off at the level of the uterine wall after the polyp has been taken out of view. Care must be taken that the pedunculated lesion is either soft and pliable enough or small enough that it can be removed through the cervix. A large pedunculated leiomyoma might be easily transected and then be very difficult to remove from the uterine cavity. Larger pedunculated lesions should be shaved into smaller portions. Leaving the lesion in the uterine cavity has been done, but it does not allow histological evaluation, is troublesome to the patient, and is less than optimal in infertility patients.

Unless they are small, sessile leiomyomas are generally not resected unless at least 40 to 50% is projecting into the uterine cavity. When less than 40 to 50% of the leiomyoma is projecting into the cavity, it becomes difficult to determine how large the remaining portion needs to be resected. Fibroids are not always round, and the depth of the intramural portion may be rather extensive (Figure 10-5). Concomitant laparoscopy is generally not used since it is neither necessary nor wise to actually resect below the level of the endometrial cavity. Perforation should not occur if this principle is not violated.

In those leiomyomas where a significant portion is intramural, a technique described by the author can be used to facilitate complete removal (Figure 10-6). In order to avoid the risk of perforation of the uterus, the leiomyoma is shaved only to the level of the uterine cavity. When the uterus is allowed to contract for the removal of the chips, the leiomyoma will be literally squeezed out of its intramural location. The author has not found it necessary to use medication to facilitate the uterus contracting. Using this technique, all of the intramural portion can usually be removed. Occasionally in very large growths, a repeat procedure may be necessary.

This process is facilitated if the edges of the fibroid, as they enter the intramural portion, are initially resected, thus "pedunculizing" the fibroid. After the extent of the intramural portion has been identified and in large part removed, that portion of the

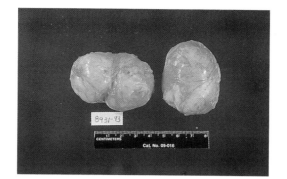

FIGURE 10-5

These leiomyoma, which were removed intact through an abdominal incision, show that the shape of leiomyoma are not always round. More may lie intramural than is apparent on hysteroscopic view. A grading scale as proposed (36) would probably correctly have identified the degree of intramural extension for the leiomyoma on the right. However, the constricted area as seen on the specimen on the left could have given the impression that the intramural portion was smaller than that projecting into the uterine cavity.

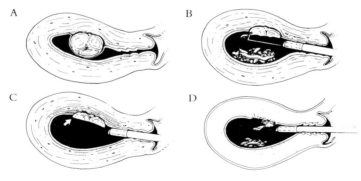

FIGURE 10-6

Removal of the intramural portion of a leiomyoma. (a) The sessile myoma before resection; (b) resection is carried down to the level of the uterine cavity; (c) each time the uterus is allowed to empty, the intramural portion is further pushed into the uterine cavity; (d) finally, the base is level with the uterine cavity and can be completely removed. (Adapted with permission from Loffer FD. Removal of large symptomatic uterine growths by the hysteroscopic resectoscope. Obstet Gynecol 1990;76:836–840.)

Removing Intrauterine Lesions: Myomectomy and Polypectomy   179 leiomyoma projecting into the cavity can then be shaved into smaller pieces.

As the intramural portion is extruded into the uterine cavity, its white, firm, and smooth capsule is readily visible and appears differently from the surrounding myometrium. The latter generally appears as crisscrossing bands of myometrium with large, open vascular channels.

When the leiomyoma is relatively large, numerous chips are created, and eventually, the resectoscope will have to be removed and the chips retrieved before the case can continue. Removal of these chips is a nuisance. Usually, a large one can be trapped against the end of the telescope by the loop electrode as the instrumentation is removed from the uterus. Polyp forceps and small curettes are then used to remove the remaining free chips. Even when the uterine cavity appears to have been completely explored, there often are numerous chips remaining.

In those patients in whom fertility is not an issue, consideration should be given to also doing an endometrial ablation. The reason for this is that other factors, such as adenomyosis, may be contributing to the heavy menstrual flow. When an endometrial ablation is done, the author prefers to use a rolling technique before the actual resection of the uterine lesion. The reasons for this are that the endometrial surface is much more easily visualized, and missed areas of ablation are less likely to occur. In addition, there are not yet any vascular spaces open, and intravasation of the distending media is much less of a problem.

RISKS

Fluid intravasation is the single greatest risk during the resection of intrauterine lesions (see Chapters 5 and 14). Some intravasation will occur with all hysteroscopic cases (42). It is increased when vascular channels are open, such as during resection procedures. Long cases will allow more fluid to intravasate than shorter cases. Excessive distending pressure will drive fluid faster into these channels. The removal of intrauterine lesions are often long cases in which numerous vascular channels are open. This predisposes these procedures to a high risk of intravasation.

The hysteroscopist has little control over the size of the lesion and the number of vascular channels that are opened. Since there is some control over the length of the procedure, the surgeon should make every effort to progress through the surgery as rapidly as is safely possible. The one factor that the surgeon has complete control over is the amount of pressure used to distend the uterus. Seventy-five mmHg pressure is quite adequate for appropriate uterine distention. Higher pressures are not necessary. They do not provide better visualization or cleaning of the uterine cavity! They do significantly increase the risks of intravasation. Since some intravasation is inevitable, strict intake and output of the low viscosity fluids used should always be maintained.

It has been the author's experience that the deficit between the fluid used and retrieved is seldom a problem when 75 mmHg pressure is used. However, if it reaches 1,000 cc, it most likely will rapidly exceed that amount. Routine electrolytes and diuretics are not necessary. When the deficit is approximately 1,500 cc, 20 mg of intravenous furosemide is given and serum electrolytes drawn. A slightly greater deficit can be accepted if mannitol is used since it has a diuretic action. Preparation should be made for the case to be brought to a conclusion even if the lesion has not been completely resected. Using these criteria, the author has not had significant problems in the four cases in which significant intravasation occurred.

Cervical lacerations occur from either the tenaculum or the dilatation of the cervix to accommodate these large-diameter instruments. Single-tooth tenacula easily tear the cervix. It is the author's preference to use a Jacob tenaculum, which secures the cervix better than a single-tooth tenaculum. Some authors use laminaria the night before the surgery to dilate the cervix, so as to avoid not only tearing the tenaculum off the cervix during dilation but also to reduce the risk of lacerating the upper cervix and lower uterine segment. Small lacerations of the cervix and lower uterine segment are commonly seen and may account for some of the intravasation experienced. However, many cervices are soft and require little dilatation. This is especially so if the patient has been bleeding heavily and passing clots. When the cervical dilation is difficult, the author prefers to use a 25 French instrument with a visual obturator (Circon ACMI). Although the loop electrode is slightly smaller, this size instrument diminishes the risk of cervical lacerations.

Perforation of the uterus should be an infrequent problem, since transection of the lesion is never carried out below the level of the uterine cavity. Perforation may occur during dilatation and entrance of the resectoscope, or if the operator becomes disoriented. Obturators are available with all sheaths and are often helpful in introducing the instruments. The resectoscope and telescope can then be introduced afterwards. The visual obturator (Circon ACMI) is especially helpful in that it allows obturation under direct visualization.

Electrical injuries are always a potential risk (43). However, they seldom occur since a continuous (cutting) waveform will have minimal spread to adjacent tissue, and injury should occur only with a perforation. Electrical injuries at the ground plate can be avoided if an REM-type system is used. Damage beyond the uterine cavity can rarely occur if the loop is not placed below the level of the uterus or advanced blindly. Therefore, most authors do not believe laparoscopic guidance should be routinely used.

Postoperative bleeding is generally not a problem. Most patients have an initial brisk and heavy flow of blood immediately following the procedure. Some of this volume is from the distending media and makes the blood loss appear greater than it actually is. Generally, the uterus quickly contracts and the bleeding slows and stops just as a postpartum uterus does. This process can be facilitated by injecting into the cervix a diluted Pitressin solution (0.3 units in 10 mL of normal saline). Foley catheters and balloons are available to tamponade the uterus, but in the author's experience, they are seldom necessary.

Postoperative adhesions in the patient desiring fertility can occur. This is probably an increased problem if two fibroids have been removed and the raw surfaces are in that position. Estrogens can be used to facilitate covering the surface if this risk appears to be high.

POSTOPERATIVE MANAGEMENT

Postoperatively, these patients will experience minimal discomfort. The need for considerable pain relief should alert the surgeon to the possibility that an intra-abdominal injury may have occurred. Usually, several oxycodene tablets are sufficient to control uterine cramping. Recovery appears to be related more to the amount of distending media intravasated and the length of the anesthesia than to any other factor. Patients are told that they can expect a bloody, watery discharge that should not be heavy. It should become progressively less over the period of time until the next menses.

RESULTS

Results of this procedure can be assessed by considering the peer review literature. There were 16 series found that gave results for the resection of leiomyomas and large polyps. Previous publications by the same authors are not included. The reason for the surgery and whether concomitant endometrial ablation was used are listed in Table 10-1. The majority of cases were done for problems of abnormal bleeding. Only a few patients were done solely because of infertility/pregnancy wastage. The exact number who had both abnormal bleeding and fertility problems was difficult to determine.

Results are listed in Table 10-2. It is difficult to obtain exact figures with which to work, since some reports do not differentiate between the results achieved by only the resection of lesions and those in which only ablation procedures were done. In addition, some authors do not state if patients were trying to become pregnant before hysteroscopic removal of the lesion or only afterward. Finally, the figures concerning results in some reports are not consistent throughout the articles. Nevertheless, uniformly very good results appear to be obtained, at least in the short term.

Pregnancy rates range from 33.3 to 66.6% of patients and the

TABLE 10-1

Indications for Removal of Intrauterine Lesions with or without Associated Endometrial Ablations

Author (ref)	No. of Cases	Indications			No. with Ablation
		AUB	Infertility	Both	
Derman (30)	108*	79	15	0	NS
Haning (12)	1	1	0	0	0
DeCherney (13)	14	14	0	0	0
Lim (16,17)	31	31	0	0	11
Hallez (18)	61	50	NS	11	0
Corson (22)	92	80	12	NS	0
Serden (23)	120	120	NS	NS	30
Indman (24)	51	51	NS	NS	38
Wortman (25)	26	26	NS	NS	22
Townsend (26)	95	95	0	0	50
Itzkowic (27)	37†	36	0	1	9
Hamou (28)	103	69	34	0	36
Pace (29)	126	108	18	0	0
Wamstecker (31)	51	39	0	12	0
Istre (32)	21	21	0	0	21
Loffer	101	86	2	13	23

AUB = abnormal uterine bleeding; NS = not stated
*Fourteen lost to follow-up
†One lost to follow-up

control of bleeding from 73.4 to 100% of patients. Bleeding failures may be immediate and result from incomplete resection or concomitant problems, such as adenomyosis. Or, they may be long-term, resulting from the same problems that occur early as well as the growth of new fibroids. Infertility patients may fail to achieve a pregnancy because of coexisting problems in addition to intrauterine lesion.

Complications experienced by those surgeons with consider-

TABLE 10-2

Successful Results Obtained Using the Resectoscope for Removal of Intrauterine Lesions

AUTHOR (REF)	INFERTILITY/ PREGNANCY WASTAGE		ABNORMAL BLEEDING	
Derman (30)	NS		73.4%	(58/79)
Haning (12)	NS		100%	(1/1)
DeCherney (13)	NS		100%	(14/14)
Lim (16,17)	0		96.7%	(30/31)
Hallez (18)	45.5%	(5/11)	93.2%	(68/73)
Corson (22)	66.6%	(8/12)	81.3%	(65/80)
Serden (23)	NS		91.6%	(98/107)
Indman (24)	NS		94.1%	(48/51)
Wortman (25)	0		95.5%	(21/22)
Townsend (26)	0		97.9%	(93/95)
Itzkowic (27)	NS		91.9%	(34/37)
Hamou (28)	55.9%	(19/34)	92.7%	(64/69)
Pace (29)	NS		90.8%	(99/101)
Wamstecker (31)	33.3%	(4/12)*	94.1%	(48/51)
Istre (32)	NS		81.0%	(17/21)*
Loffer	46.6%	(7/15)	74.7%	(71/95)
Total	51.2%	(43/84)	88.6%	(829/935)

NS = not stated
*Estimated exact figures were not given

able experience have been few, indicating this can be a safe procedure for patients (Table 10-3). The risk of excessive fluid intravasation always exists. The literature contains many reports (42), and many others are never reported. Strict intake and output of distending media must be maintained. Occasional perforation of the uterus during dilation, insertion of the scope, or retrieval of chips may occur. Perforation with an activated electrode should be very

TABLE 10-3

Complications Occurring with the Resectoscope for the Removal of Intrauterine Lesions

Author (Ref)	No. of Cases	Excess Fluid Absorption	Uterus Perforation	Electric Injury	Bleeding	Infection	Resulting Lap
Derman (30)	108	0	0	0	4	0	2
Haning (12)	1	0	0	0	0	0	0
DeCherney (13)	14	0	0	0	0	0	0
Lim (16,17)	31	0	0	0	0	0	0
Hallez (18)	61	0	1	0	0	0	1
Corson (22)	92	0	3	0	1	1	0
Serden (23)	120	1	1	0	4	2	0
Indman (24)	51	2	0	0	1	0	0
Wortman (25)	26	0	0	0	2	0	0
Townsend (26)	95	0	0	0	0	0	0
Itzkowic (27)	37	1	0	0	8	1	1
Hamou (28)	103	NS	NS	NS	NS	NS	NS
Pace (29)	126	0	0	0	1	0	0
Wamstecker (31)	51	0	1	0	0	0	0
Loffer	101	4	1	0	0	0	0
Total	1071	9	7	0	21	4	4

NS = not stated

uncommon. The risk of serious bleeding requiring some management, such as with an intrauterine balloon, occurred in only 2.2% of cases. Transfusions were generally not necessary.

Long-term results are available from only two series. The longest follow-up covered 94 patients who had undergone submucous fibroid resection (30). Late problems, primarily persistent or recurrent bleeding, occurred in 24.5% of patients; however, further surgery was required in only 15.9% of patients. No further surgery was required after 9 years of follow-up in 83.9% of patients.

The second series with long-term follow-up is the author's. It is based on the use of the resectoscope to remove large symptomatic intrauterine lesions since 1984. Some of the cases described here have been previously published (21). In reviewing the first 101 patients, 86 were done for abnormal bleeding, two for infertility, and 13 for both infertility and associated abnormal bleeding. Eighty lesions were fibroids and 21 were large polyps (Table 10-4). Table 10-5 shows the results achieved for this group of patients. Both of the patients who had been infertile became pregnant and successfully delivered as did five of the 13 who had both infertility and heavy bleeding. Four of the 99 patients with heavy bleeding were followed less than 6 months. Heavy bleeding was controlled in all but 12 of the 95 patients with that problem who were followed longer than 6 months. Of the 12 patients whose bleeding was not totally controlled by this procedure, five had a repeat myoma resection, two had an endometrial ablation, and three underwent hyster-

TABLE 10-4

Lesions Treated by Resectoscope

	ABNORMAL UTERINE BLEEDING	INFERTILITY	BOTH
No. of Patients	86	2	13
Fibroid	66	2	12
Polyp	20	0	1

TABLE 10-5

Resectoscope Results

	ABNORMAL UTERINE BLEEDING	INFERTILITY	BOTH
Total No. of Patients	86*	2	13
Pregnancy	2	2	5
AUB – controlled w/o ablation	48*	NA	12
controlled with ablation	23	NA	NA
failed w/o ablation	11	NA	1
failed with ablation	0	NA	NA
Hyst – w/o ablation	5	0	2
with ablation	1	NA	NA
Follow-up less than 6 months	4	0	0

AUB = abnormal uterine bleeding; Hyst = hysterectomy
*One asymptomatic large polyp found at CAT scan in a 65-year-old patient

ectomy. Two patients had enough benefit that they elected to have no further surgery.

Early in the author's series, it was his practice in patients with abnormal bleeding to remove only the intrauterine lesion. The rationale for this approach was based on the belief that the intrauterine lesion was causing the problem and the least surgery done to correct the problem was the appropriate course to take. However, a review of 12 patients who had continued or recurrent bleeding problems showed that this might not be the best approach. One developed a new fibroid, six had continued growth of a partially resected fibroid, and one had adenomyosis. The cause of continued abnormal bleeding was not known in the two patients undergoing a later ablation or in the two patients who refused further therapy. These problems may not have occurred if these patients had had a concomitant ablation. Table 10-6 shows that, thus far, none of the patients with the concomitant ablation have failed because of bleeding problems, whereas 17% without ablation failed.

TABLE 10-6

Long-term Effectiveness after Initial Surgery of Controlling AUB by Submucous Fibroid Resection with and without Endometrial Ablation

	No. of Patients	Success	Failure
Without ablation	72	60 (83%)	12 (17%)
With ablation	23	23 (100%)	0
Total*	95		

*Follow-up greater than 6 months

Only three of the eight patients who have come to hysterectomy in the author's series were having abnormal bleeding (Table 10-7). These three elected to have hysterectomy rather than repeat hysteroscopic procedures. One had developed a new fibroid, one prolapsed a partially resected fibroid, and one had adenomyosis and an intramural fibroid. Two of the patients who had a hysterectomy had their resectoscope procedure for both infertility and abnormal bleeding. One never became pregnant but had no further abnormal bleeding. Her hysterectomy was apparently done because of the presence of asymptomatic subserosal fibroids. The other patient had endometriosis surgery following her fibroid resection before becoming pregnant. She was having normal menses but underwent a hysterectomy for pelvic pain after her delivery. Three other patients who were having normal menses had a hysterectomy for pain. One patient had pelvic adhesions and two had adenomyosis. One of these latter patients had had a concomitant ablation done with her resection. All of the three patients who had further problems with bleeding and one of those with pain may have had their hysterectomies prevented by concomitant ablation.

In reviewing the author's (as well as other) case series reports, it is clear that those patients presenting with infertility or pregnancy wastage are frequently helped, although there are often coexisting

TABLE 10-7

Age of Patient at Initial Surgery and Length of Time to and Reason for Hysterectomy

	AGE (YEARS)	MO
Asymptomatic fibroids*	38	13
AUB		
recurrent fibroid	41	12
fibroid + adenomyosis	42	14
prolapsed fibroid	46	6
Pain		
adenomyosis	38	47
adenomyosis	39	33
adhesionosis	38	33
endometriosis†	33	40

AUB = abnormal uterine bleeding
*Patient with AUB and infertile who never became pregnant
†Was infertile with AUB before resection and became pregnant after endometriosis surgery

factors. Menorrhagia is controlled in the majority of patients, but since the uterus remains, a failure rate can be expected and patients should be aware of this.

After reviewing the long-term results of his own series, the author has concluded that concomitant ablation in those patients not desiring fertility may significantly improve the results obtained in controlling bleeding. The benefits may result from constricting the cavity, thus decreasing the chance of further submucous fibroid growth. It may also improve the results in those patients who have adenomyosis. The author has further concluded that those patients in whom pain is a significant component of their problem are probably not well served by undergoing resection with or without an ablation since only the discomfort of the passage of blood clots can be guaranteed to be controlled.

CLINICAL PEARLS

✖ Most submucous myomas and clinically significant endometrial polyps are not identified by blind procedures, such as a D & C or endometrial biopsy.

✖ Patients without significant dysmenorrhea should understand their pain may not be helped by removal of the polyp or fibroid.

✖ Although the risk of malignancy is low, tissue removed should always undergo pathological evaluation.

✖ Resection of myoma should not be carried below the level of the uterine cavity.

✖ The intramural portion can frequently be completely removed by allowing the uterus to contract and, thus, project the remaining part of the myoma into the cavity.

✖ Resectoscopic removal of submucous myomas may be accomplished by significant fluid intravasation.

more valuable the closer patients are to menopause, since there are fewer years for the risks of increasing bleeding and pain to develop.

REFERENCES

1. Loffer FD. Hysteroscopy with selective endometrial sampling compared with D&C for abnormal uterine bleeding: the value of a negative hysteroscopic view. Obstet Gynecol 1989;73:16–20.
2. Gimpleson RJ, Rappold HO. A comparative study between panoramic hysteroscopy with directed biopsies and dilatation and curettage. Am J Obstet Gynecol 1988;158:489–492.
3. Kessler I, Lancet M. Hysterography and hysteroscopy: a comparison. Fertil Steril 1984;46:709–710.

4. Snowden EU, Jarrett JC II, Dagwood MY. Comparison of diagnostic accuracy of laparoscopy, hysteroscopy and hysterosalpingography in evaluation of female infertility. Fertil Steril 1984;41:708–713.

5. Valle RF, Sciarra JJ. Current status of hysteroscopy in gynecologic practice. Fertil Steril 1979;32:619–632.

6. Fedele L, Bianchi S, Dorta M, Brioschi D, Zanotti F, Vercellini P. Transvaginal ultrasonography versus hysteroscopy in the diagnosis of uterine submucous myomas. Obstet Gynecol 1991;77:745–748.

7. Goldstein SR, Nachtigall M, Snyder JR, Nachtigall L. Endometrial assessment by vaginal ultrasonography before endometrial sampling in patients with postmenopausal bleeding. Am J Obstet Gynecol 1990;163:119–123.

8. Randolph JR, Ying YK, Maier DB, Schmidt CL, Riddick DH. Comparison of real-time ultrasonography, hystosalpingography, and laparoscopy/hysteroscopy in the evaluation of uterine abnormalities and tubal patency. Fertil Steril 1986;46:828–832.

9. Norment WB, Sikes, Berry FX, Bird I. Hysteroscopy. In: Turcle R, ed. Surg Clin North Am Chicago: WB Saunders, 1957:1377–1386.

10. Neuwirth RS, Amin HK. Excision of submucous fibroids with hysteroscopic control. Am J Obstet Gynecol 1976;126:95–99.

11. Neuwirth RS. A new technique for an additional experience with hysteroscopic resection of submucous fibroids. Am J Obstet Gynecol 1978;131:91–94.

12. Haning RV, Harkins PG, Uehling DT. Preservation of fertility by transcervical resection of a benign mesodermal uterine tumor with the resectoscope and glycine distending media. Fertil Steril 1980; 33:209–210.

13. DeCherney AH, Polan ML. Hysteroscopic management of intrauterine lesions and intractable uterine bleeding. Obstet Gynecol 1983; 61:392–397.

14. Neuwirth RS. Hysteroscopic management of symptomatic submucous fibroids. Am J Obstet Gynecol 1983;62:509–511.

15. Loffer FD. Hysteroscopic management of menorrhagia. Acta Eur Fertil 1986;17:463–465.

16. Lin BL, Miyamoto N, Aoki R, Iwata Y. Transcervical resection of submucous myoma. Acta Obstet Gynecol Jpn 1986;38:1647–1652.

17. Lin BL, Miyamoto N, Tomomater M, et al. The development of a new hysteroscopic resectoscope and its clinical applications on trans-

cervical resection (TCR) and endometrial ablation (EA). Jap J Obstet Gynecol Endoscopy 1988;4:56–61.

18. Hallez JP, Netter A, Cartier R. Methodical intrauterine resection. Am J Obstet Gynecol 1987;156:1080–1084.

19. Hallez JP, Perino A. Endoscopic intrauterine resection: principles and technique. Acta Eur Fertil 1988;19:17–21.

20. Brooks PG, Loffer FD, Serden SP. Resectoscopic removal of symptomatic intrauterine lesions. J Reprod Med 1989;34:435–437.

21. Loffer FD. Removal of large symptomatic intrauterine growths by the hysteroscopic resectoscope. Obstet Gynecol 1990;76:836–840.

22. Corson SL, Brooks PG. Resectoscopic myomectomy. Fertil Steril 1991;55:1041–1044.

23. Serden SP, Brooks PG. Treatment of abnormal uterine bleeding with the gynecologic resectoscope. J Reprod Med 1991;36:676–679.

24. Indman PD. Hysteroscopic treatment of menorrhagia associated with uterine leiomyomas. Obstet Gynecol 1993;81:716–720.

25. Wortman M, Daggett A. Hysteroscopic management of intractable uterine bleeding. A review of 103 cases. J Reprod Med 1991;38:505–510.

26. Townsend DE, Fields G, McCausland A, Kauffman K. Diagnostic and operative hysteroscopy in the management of persistent postmenopausal bleeding. Obstet Gynecol 1993;82:419–421.

27. Itzkowic D. Submucous fibroids: clinical profile and hysteroscopic management. Aust NZ J Obstet Gynecol 1993;33:63–67.

28. Hamou J. Electroresection of fibroids. In: Sutton CJG, Diamond M, eds. Endoscopic surgery for gynecologists London: WB Saunders, 1993:327–330.

29. Pace S. Transcervical resection of benign endocavitary lesions. Gynecol Endosc 1993;2:165–169.

30. Derman SG, Rehnstrom J, Neuwirth RS. The long-term effectiveness of hysteroscopic treatment of menorrhagia and leiomyomas. Obstet Gynecol 1991;77:591–594.

31. Wamstecker K, Emanual MH, deKruix JH. Transcervical hysteroscopic resection of submucous fibroids for abnormal uterine bleeding: results regarding the degree of intramural extension. Obstet Gynecol 1993;32:736–740.

32. Istre O, Skajaa K, Holm-Nielsen P, Forman A. The second-look ap-

pearance of the uterine cavity after resection of the endometrium. Gynecol Endoscopy 1993;2:159–163.

33. Wamstecker K, deBlok S. Diagnostic hysteroscopy: technique and documentation. In: Sutton CJH, Diamond M, eds. Endoscopic surgery for gynecologists. London: WB Saunders, 1993;263–276.

34. Emanuel MH, Wamsteker K, Eastham WN, Kroeks MVAM. Leiomyosarcoma or cellular leiomyoma diagnosed after hysteroscopical transcervical resection of a presumed leiomyoma. Gynecol Endoscopy 1992;1:161–164.

35. Valle RF. Hysteroscopic removal of submucous leiomyomas. J Gynecol Surg 1990;6:89–96.

36. Dequesne J, DeGrandi P. Focal treatment of uterine bleeding and infertility with Nd:YAG laser and flexible hysteroscope. Gynecol Surg 1989;5:177–182.

37. Baggish MS, Sze EHM, Morgan G. Hysteroscopic treatment of symptomatic submucous myomata uteri with the Nd:YAG laser. J Gynecol surg 1989;5:27–36.

38. Donnez J, Gillerst S, Bourgonjon D, Clerckx F, Nisolle M. Neodymium:YAG laser hysteroscopy in large submucous fibroids. Fertil Steril 1990;54:999–1003.

39. McLucas B. Diathermy polyp snare: a new modality for treatment of myomas and polyps. Gynecol Endosc 1992;1:107–110.

40. Goldrath MH. Vaginal removal of the pedunculated submucous myoma: the use of laminaria. Obstet Gynecol 1987;70:670–672.

41. McCausland VM, Fields GA, McCausland AM, Townsend DE. Tubo-ovarian abscesses after operative hysteroscopy. J Reprod Med 1993;38:198–200.

42. Loffer FD. Complications from uterine distention. In: Corfman RS, Diamond MP, DeCherney AL, eds. Complications of laparascopy and hysteroscopy. Boston: Blackwell Scientific Publications, 1993: 177–186.

43. Sullivan B, Kenney P, Seibel M. Hysteroscopic resection of fibroid with thermal injury to sigmoid. Obstet Gynecol 1992;80:546–547.

11

Control of Menorrhagia by Electrodesiccation

Thierry G. Vancaillie

Destruction of the endometrium by any method of energy transfer is commonly called *ablation*. Ablation can be understood as destruction as well as removal of tissue. Recently, the term *resection* has been introduced, when the electrical loop is used to actually resect the endometrium. Since then, ablation is perceived as being opposite to resection; it is not. Ablation could be said to entail the possibility of resection.

For the purpose of avoiding confusion, the term ablation will be avoided and replaced with *electrodesiccation* when relating to a method involving the resectoscope with a large electrode. *Ablation* will only be used as a generic term encompassing any method of in vivo destruction or removal of the endometrium.

Surgical treatment (other than hysterectomy) for excessive uterine bleeding has not been part of medical textbooks. However, attempts at conservative surgical treatment of menorrhagia are not new at all. In fact, in our modern literature, we can trace such reports back to the first two decades of this century (1).

Without going into detailed philosophical discussions of why alternative methods of treating abnormal uterine bleeding are more or less widespread, it may be said that the current impetus for uterus-sparing surgical treatment is due to greater involvement of the patient in making medical decisions.

INDICATIONS

Abnormal uterine bleeding caused by a benign condition is a generic denomination of the indications for endometrial ablation. However, the true indication for this procedure is menorrhagia, i.e., excessive menstrual bleeding without disruption of the cycle.

The objective of the procedure is cytoreduction of the endometrium, which will reduce the amount of blood flow but not influence the timing.

Combination treatments involving other intrauterine surgical procedures, such as myomectomy, can be considered when dealing with clinical conditions other than menorrhagia.

Currently, there is not sufficient knowledge about the uterine microanatomy and the effect this has on the type of surgery to be performed. Can the surgeon visually recognize such conditions as adenomyosis? Is it preferable to desiccate or resect the adenomyotic tissue? These are among the questions still unanswered.

Endometrial ablation brings along beneficial side effects. Along with the reduction in menstrual flow, there seems to be a reduction in dysmenorrhea and even premenstrual syndrome (2) symptomatology. Neither one of these conditions, however, can be considered an indication for endometrial ablation. It also seems important to mention that if a patient complains of pelvic pain, an effort should be made to characterize the pain more precisely. One cannot just assume that the pain will be improved after the procedure. In some cases, de novo pelvic pain presents a new challenge to the treating physician.

Patients with known endometriosis, for example, will more than likely not be satisfied. There is no reason to believe that endometrial ablation will affect the pathophysiologic process of pelvic pain related to endometriosis. The question of whether a combination of laparoscopic resection of endometriosis and endometrial ablation is an acceptable alternative to hysterectomy is out of the realm of this chapter. This approach is technically feasible, and, in my opinion, an acceptable alternative in well-informed patients who desire to conserve their reproductive organs—and who take responsibility for this decision.

Sterility is another potential side effect of endometrial ablation. However, endometrial ablation cannot be considered a method of sterilization because endometrial tissue may remain, and pregnancies have been reported. The pregnancy rate after endometrial ablation is low as far as we know, but figures are guesses rather than exact numbers.

One aspect of endometrial ablation with regard to sterilization should be emphasized: endometrial ablation might be the only method of female sterilization with a physiologic indicator of success, namely amenorrhea.

METHODS

Electrodesiccation of the endometrium is achieved using large monopolar electrodes. Originally, a 2-mm ball electrode was inserted into the uterus blindly and activated while the surgeon moved the probe within the uterine cavity (1). This rather crude technique was successful in arresting menorrhagia in an emergency room setup in the majority of cases.

Currently, the resectoscope is the method of choice for electrodesiccation of the endometrium. The decisions to be made are which electrode to choose and what settings on the electrosurgical unit are ideal.

The electrodes available are spherical or variations thereof. The objectives to be achieved are good contact with the tissue at varying angles and large contact area to lower the power density. A low power density is required to obtain desiccation and not fulguration. Sharp edges or uninsulated branches are to be avoided. These edges are sites that can easily lead to sparking between the electrode and the tissue. When sparking occurs, there are two detrimental coexisting effects. The first one is that the power density of electrical current at other sites of the electrode will be reduced to a level ineffective in producing desiccation. The second effect is that sparking will cause carbonization of the tissue hit by the spark. The impedance of that tissue will greatly increase and, thereby, prevent destruction by electrodesiccation of the deeper layers.

In summary, the choice of electrode should be dictated by the following factors (Figure 11-1):

1. Spherical, ellipsoid shape or any variation of it.
2. Smooth conductive surface, noncorroded, i.e., unused.
3. No edges or sharp angles.
4. Intact insulation.
5. Approximately 3 mm in diameter; a larger contact area may require a high output electrosurgical unit.

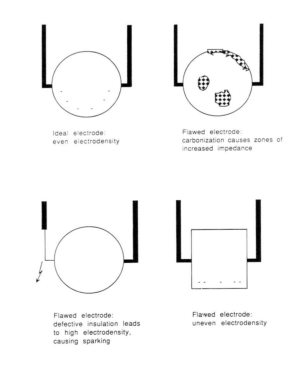

Ideal electrode:
even electrodensity

Flawed electrode:
carbonization causes zones of
increased impedance

Flawed electrode:
defective insulation leads
to high electrodensity,
causing sparking

Flawed electrode:
uneven electrodensity

FIGURE 11-1

Graphical representation of the ideal electrode and the possible defects.

198   **Gynecologic Resectoscopy**

The discussion on what type of current and what settings to use on the electrosurgical unit is found in the section on "Surgical Technique."

PREOPERATIVE MANAGEMENT

A thorough history and physical examination are obvious prerequisites. It should be made clear that, although an endometrial ablation is a uterus-sparing procedure, there should be no further desire for pregnancy.

Laboratory values of the serum electrolytes should be considered in advance so that possible abnormalities can be dealt with prior to surgery. This is especially important in patients with systemic disorders affecting the electrolyte balance, such as liver and kidney diseases. Patients receiving diuretics should be given potassium replacement if they do not use it already. Careful evaluation of the coagulation parameters is obtained in patients with a thromboembolic disorder or on anticoagulant therapy. Abnormal studies are not necessarily a contraindication for endometrial ablation, but they will require a personalized approach to management of intra- and postoperative risk of bleeding.

Histology of the endometrium is obtained in every patient either at the time of the procedure or in advance. Patients at risk for adenocarcinoma of the endometrium should undergo an endometrial biopsy or hysteroscopy and biopsy prior to scheduling of the ablation. The patient at risk for developing endometrial cancer, such as the diabetic patient and the patient with polycystic ovary disease, should be counseled very carefully. An effort should be made to explain the risk-benefit ratio of vaginal hysterectomy versus ablation.

Hormonal preparation of the endometrium is indicated in selected cases. The objective of the hormonal manipulation is to perform the surgery at a time that the endometrium is reduced to the basal layer. This occurs naturally during menses or in the early postpartum. However, to ensure that a patient will indeed present with an atrophic endometrium, the use of gonadotropin agonists is indicated. This is critical when ablation is performed using an electrodesiccation technique as opposed to resection. When resecting, the sugeon can visually assure that the entire endometrial lining is removed. When desiccating, there is no such visual end-point. The latter method will, therefore, be effective only when the endometrium is thin. This can be achieved reliably only with medication, such as Lupron depot (TAP pharmaceutical Deerfield, Ill).

Patients in whom a desiccation technique is definitively preferred over resection are the individuals with coagulopathies, endogenic or iatrogenic, and in whom fluid overload is to be avoided at all cost because of reduced renal function. Some patients without systemic condition may also benefit from preparation with Lupron. They are the patients in whom ultrasonography has indicated the presence of a highly grown endometrium. In such cases, desiccation is not feasible, and resection may be quite tedious. Preoperative reduction of the bulk of the endometrial tissue will facilitate the procedure and, therefore, also increase the chances of success. The indications for hormonal suppression of the endometrium should be set liberally early in someone's experience because the use of these agents greatly facilitates the procedure.

SURGICAL TECHNIQUE

The patient is positioned in lithotomy with legs in stirrups. Use of candycane-type stirrups is indicated because of the increased mobility provided to the surgeon with regard to manipulation of the endoscope.

Local anesthesia in the form of a paracervical block combined with systemic analgesia is adequate for almost every modality of operative hysteroscopy. Conduction anesthesia or general endotracheal anesthesia are excellent alternatives. Application of a paracervical block may be used even if the patient is under general anesthesia since the block will also suppress postoperative pain. This is even more pronounced when long-lasting anesthetics, such as bupivacaine, are used.

Admixture of Pitressin to the local anesthetic has the additional benefit of reducing blood flow during the procedure. This is advantageous when performing a resection technique. When only desiccation is used, there may not be any benefit. The impact of Pitressin on fluid absorption is unclear.

Cervical dilation is performed using any of the established techniques. The use of KY gel appears to smoothen the dilatation process. In addition, waiting until the paracervical block is well established seems to have a beneficial effect on the cervical dilation process. Cervical lacerations are a real problem because fluid absorption through these lacerations can take dramatic proportions very quickly. When a cervical laceration is noted, the surgeon should take extra precautions in obtaining accurate estimates of the fluid deficit.

The cervix is dilated to Hegar 10. This will allow smooth maneuverability of the endoscope during the procedure. Indeed, it is important that insertion and extraction of the endoscope through the endocervical canal do not require force. This would lead to jerky movements and inaccuracy of the surgical manipulation. Over-dilatation had been advocated by some to increase the flow of distention medium. Continuous flow resectoscopes have channels that are quite sufficient in diameter to carry the medium in and out. Smooth maneuverability of the endoscope is the one priority.

Some surgeons perform suction and evacuation of the uterus prior to electrodesiccation of the endometrium, even in cases where the endometrium was hormonally suppressed. They do this in order to ensure that there is a histologic specimen.

The fully assembled resectoscope is then introduced into the uterine cavity. This can be done under direct vision or with an obturator. Direct vision is what the author prefers because this is the only time early in the procedure where the operator has a chance to visually inspect the cervical canal and detect lacerations, a cause for concern. In addition, blind and forceful insertion of the resectoscope, using the obturator, may lead to uterine perforation.

The irrigation system is set in place. A pump-driven system with a pressure measurement device can be used. Simple gravity with large bore tubing ("TUR" tubing) is equally adequate. The latter is the system I favor. It is important to have a method for optimal collection of the irrigant. Either the circulating nurse or the anesthesiologist is in charge of calculating the difference between inflow and outflow. This seems easy and straightforward but it is not! The main culprit for discordances between calculated difference and true difference is the lack of a watertight continuous flow system. The difficult part is the collection of fluid spilled along the resectoscope, within the vagina, and on to the operating table and floor. The patient should be draped in such a way to allow the fluid to be collected from underneath the buttocks into a funnel, which is then connected to the collection canister. Too often a 1-L canister is used; it will have to be replaced so rapidly that there is no time left for calculating the difference between in and out. Simplification of this irrigation setup is a high priority. One of many possibilities is to use 3-Liter irrigation fluid bags on a high pole and six 3-L aspiration canisters arranged in series. The aspirated fluid will automatically flow over to the next canister when one is full. The empty fluid bags are left hanging on the pole so that a quick scan of the number of empty bags and full canisters will give the surgeon a rough idea of the fluid overload. There is ample room for modification of such a system. The objectives are to retrieve as much fluid as possible and to be able to calculate the difference quickly.

The uterine cavity is then carefully inspected. In particular, the surgeon identifies the tubal ostia, detects and characterizes intrauterine lesions, and looks for scars left by cesarean section and other uterine surgery. Unless the anatomy is carefully assessed, the procedure should not commence. At this time, the surgeon selects the type of electrode best suited for the particular procedure to be performed. For novices, it is recommended to start with the large ball- or barrel-type electrodes. The choice of electrode will primarily depend on the pathology present. An intrauterine tumor, such as a fibroid, has to be resected with a loop-type electrode. The surgeon may elect to proceed with resection of the remaining endometrium rather than electrodesiccation. However, it is certainly not wrong to perform the electrodesiccation first and to resect the fibroid later. It is my experience that marking the fundus and ostial areas with the ball electrode helps in subsequent orientation.

Systematic is the buzz word in electrodesiccation of the endometrium. Each and every surgeon has to determine the sequence in which the endometrial surface will be desiccated. The author begins at the fundus, drawing a line between both ostia. Then, the electrode is rolled over the anterior wall first and progressed clockwise. Some fine tuning may be required at the level of the ostia and the internal cervical os. A second pass is not required.

Choice and application of electrical current could be the subject of a book on its own. There is appreciable variation among the different electrosurgical units available in the operating room. Making recommendations is, therefore, somewhat hazardous. As a surgeon, I like to choose the settings on the unit according to clinically observable results. These visual end points are typical and reproducible. The settings on particular electrosurgical units will be widely variable for identical clinical results. Therefore, I will not express recommendations for a particular unit nor the brand name of any equipment.

The electrodesiccation process can be divided into two steps (Figure 11-2): (1) the initiation phase and (2) dynamic phase. During the initiation phase, the electrode is brought in contact with the surface of the endometrial cavity. Contact is firmly achieved before current is established. Following contact, the surgeon keys the pedal, thereby activating the electrode. Optimal current settings will result in immediate blanching of the tissue in contact with the electrode. This area of blanching slowly spreads circumferential around the electrode. Small gas vacuoles ("bubbles") are seen arising from the tissues around the blanched area. Larger vacuoles form within the blanched tissue. If sparking or tissue disintegration is observed, the settings are too high. A continuous sinusoidal (cutting) waveform is better than a damped (coagulation) waveform, provided that sufficient voltage is available to drive the current through a highly impeding tissue, such as partly desiccated endometrium. During the dynamic phase of the procedure, the electrode is painstakingly slowly rolled or dragged over the surface of the

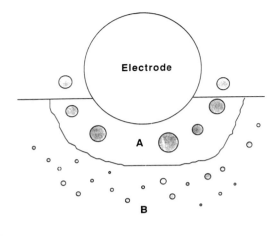

A: Tissue damage zone with visible blanching and large vacuoles

B: Tissue damage zone with small vacuoles

FIGURE 11-2

Graphical representation of the visual control of the electrodesiccation process.

uterine cavity. The pressure on the electrode is firmly maintained while moving the instrument. The desiccation artifacts earlier described will remain visible. Vacuolization and blanching of tissue have to be observed in front of the electrode. These phenomena are the only clinical data available to the surgeon to use in estimating the adequacy of electrodesiccation. Depth of tissue destruction is not visible per se. However, when tissue is seen blanching in front of the electrode, one may safely assume that tissue underneath the electrode will also be affected.

Carbonization of either the tissue or the electrode has to be avoided. A new electrode should be used for each procedure because the metal will be affected by usage and carry current less effectively. A carbonized electrode requires increasing the power setting and will, therefore, likely cause sparking between the electrode and the tissue in an effort to bridge the gap created by the carbon deposit on the surface of the electrode. This sparking will, in turn, dry out the surface of the tissue too rapidly, thereby preventing desiccation of the deeper layers. Carbonization of the tissue has a similar negative effect on the depth of tissue destruction. The most likely cause of carbonization is the use of excessive electrical power.

In summary, the lowest effective power setting is the ideal setting. A low power will require slow motion of the electrode, which will lead to deep desiccation of the endomyometrial tissue. It is recommended that the surgeon use the same generator for these procedures in order to develop expertise with that particular unit. This, in turn, increases the likelihood of positive outcome.

Slow and systematic electrodesiccation of all endometrial surfaces is recommended. Repeat passages of the electrode over the surface do not replace the efficiency of a single slow and systematic approach. Partially desiccated tissue, resulting from a rapid pass with the electrode, will present increased impedance to the electrode during the next pass. This increased impedance may prevent all further heat generation in the tissue. Adequate ablation may not be obtained.

Lesions, such as fibroids within the cavity, represent a challenge. The rigid equipment commonly used for operative hysteroscopy limits the accessibility of areas within the cavity that are masked by the intrauterine mass. Either the surgeon accepts that the ablative procedure will be incomplete, or the mass is resected at least partially to allow the ablative procedure to be complete. I believe the surgeon who engages in operative hysteroscopy should be versed in the use of all different electrodes and attachments that are available. An effort should be made to resect the intrauterine mass in addition to the electrodesiccation of the endometrium. Ideally, ultrasonography has been performed prior to the ablation in order to avoid embarrassing moments for the surgeon.

When desiccating the endomyometrial surface, the endometrium has a tendency to detach from the underlying myometrium. This should be of no concern to the operator. In some instances, the strips of tissue detaching are of varying thickness and the exposed myometrial surface is irregular. This shows that the endometrium-myometrium interface is irregular. This clinical observation most likely correlates with adenomyosis. It is, as of yet, unclear whether this finding should lead to alteration in surgical technique or patient management.

RISKS

Risks associated with operative hysteroscopy are fluid overload, bleeding, and infection. Subsequent pregnancy is not a risk per se because the procedure is not intended for sterilization purposes.

Fluid overload is of primary concern. Careful measurement of inflow and outflow is essential when performing operative hysteroscopy. Simple schemes to increase the speed by which the difference between in- and outflow can be measured are important. As mentioned before, one of these simple schemes is to use 3-L bags for irrigation and 3-L canisters for recuperation of fluids. This allows the surgeon, at any time, to quickly estimate the amount of fluid not accounted for.

The choice of irrigation fluid is determined by electrical conductivity and osmolality. Nonconductive fluids are to be used with electrosurgery. This is not because the presence of electrolytes would burn the patient but because the electrolytes diffuse the current and thereby drastically reduce the power density. As a result, very little heat is generated in the tissues to be destroyed.

The osmolality of fluid is determined by the number of particles in the fluid (3). The effects of fluids on distribution of water in the body are dependent on the permeability of cell and capillary membranes for the various particles present in the fluid.

The commonly used irrigation fluids are composed of water with particles that readily diffuse through the capillary membrane but not through the cell membrane. Therefore, infusion of these fluids will cause water redistribution in the entire extracellular compartment (EC). The intracellular compartment (IC) will be indirectly affected by the dilutional effects on the concentration of solutes (principally Na^+) in the EC. The IC will maintain the transmembranous gradient of concentrations of Na^+ and K^+ through active pumping. This process will result in intracellular low K^+ concentration and swelling due to absorption of water in the cell. Clinically, this *water intoxication* manifests itself by cerebral edema (confusion, drowsiness, coma, and death). Acute dilutional hyponatremia is synonymous with water intoxication.

One-half of body weight represents total body fluid. Extracellular (intravascular and interstitial) fluid equals 45% of total body fluid.

Table 11-1 demonstrates the effect that one liter of overload is sufficient to bring a normonatremic patient in the abnormal range!

Table 11-2 shows the same example when there is a 3-L overload. This will decrease the patient's sodium to 120 meq/L, which is the level at which symptoms of cerebral edema may appear. In addition, the symptoms of cerebral edema will be masked by general anesthesia. Management of fluid overload has been discussed in Chapter 5.

TABLE 11-1

The Effects of One Liter Fluid Overload

80 kg patient
Total body water (TB) = 40 L
EC = 40 × 0.45 = 18 L
Total Na^+ = 18 × 140 meq/L = 2520 meq
Fluid overload of 1 L of electrolyte-free solution
New EC = 19 L
New $[Na^+]$ = 2520/19 = 132.6 meq/L

TABLE 11-2

The Effects of Three Liter Fluid Overload

80 kg patient
Fluid overload of 3 L of electrolyte-free solution
New EC = 21 L
New $[Na^+]$ = 2520/21 = 120 meq/L

Bleeding is a rare complication of electrodesiccation of the endometrium. Generally, it will be due to either cervical laceration or uterine perforation. Hemorrhagic complications are more likely to occur with the loop electrode during myoma or endometrial resection of a fibroid or of the endometrium. Management of hemorrhagic complications will depend on the location of the source of bleeding and the severity of the condition. Uterine bleeding, when visualized under hysteroscopic view, can be stopped using the ball-end electrode. The electrode is firmly applied to the bleeding area. A low wattage continuous ("cutting") current is then applied for one to two minutes. This will lead to coaptation of the bleeding source and control of the hemorrhage. Diffuse bleeding from the cavity can be controlled with insertion of a balloon (Foley catheter with 30 cc bulb). The balloon is inflated with 10 to 20 cc of fluid until firm resistance is perceived. Methergine can be given IV to stimulate myometrial contractions, thereby increasing the tamponading force. The balloon is gradually deflated, e.g., 50% of its volume every two hours, until it can be removed by gentle traction. Leaving the balloon in the uterine cavity for more than 24 hours is not recommended. Antibiotic coverage is added to the treatment for the duration of the tamponade, and the patient is kept in observation for at least 23 hours.

Infectious complications were the only complications initially reported in 1937 by surgeons performing endometrial electrodesiccation (1). The incidence of endomyometritis and subsequent pelvic abscess was 3%. Some of these patients went on to develop fistulas between the uterus and small bowel! Therefore, the threat of serious infectious complications is real. The clinical manifestations of postoperative endomyometritis are hemorrhage, pain, and fever. None of these symptoms needs to be dramatic to raise the suspicion of infection. When a patient presents with increasingly heavier vaginal bleeding in the early days after the procedure, treatment for endomyometritis should be initiated even in the absence of fever. Treatment consists of high-dose broad spectrum antibiotics, which can be given on an outpatient basis. Hospitalization is required only in severe cases. Patients unresponsive to antibiotic treatment should undergo hysterectomy. A prolonged "wait and see" attitude may be detrimental to the patient because endomyometritis may quickly degenerate into a fulminating sepsis and subsequent demise of the patient. Fortunately, infection rarely occurs (4).

Pregnancy is not a true complication of the procedure but should be discussed with the patient. The incidence of pregnancy after endometrial ablation is, in fact, unknown. A compilation of a large number of procedures yielded the figure of 1% incidence of pregnancy, mostly intrauterine, after endometrial ablation (5). Patients at risk for pregnancy after ablation should be advised to use some method of contraception or deal with the prospect of possibly undergoing a pregnancy interruption.

POSTOPERATIVE MANAGEMENT

The immediate postoperative management consists of monitoring of vital signs at regular intervals. Vaginal bleeding should not exceed the amount that can be expected after procedures, such as a D & C.

Pain, in the form of cramping, is common. When a paracervical block has been used, this pain is minimal. Otherwise, the uterine cramping during the first two hours following the procedure can be severe and require sedation with drugs such as morphine or meperidine (Demerol). Pain requiring sedation that persists for several hours should alert the physician that a complication has occurred, related to inadvertent heat damage to neighboring organs.

Postoperative hormonal treatment has been shown to increase the proportion of patients with amenorrhea (5). However, the combined incidence of amenorrhea and hypomenorrhea remains unchanged. Depo Provera is the drug most commonly used because it is conveniently administered only once, in the immediate postoperative period.

Prophylactic antibiotics are given by some. It has not been demonstrated that this reduces the incidence of infectious complications.

The first postoperative visit is scheduled approximately one week after the procedure. The blood-tinged vaginal discharge has by that time usually ceased. On physical examination, the uterus should feel firm. Persistent or increasing blood-tinged discharge and/or uterine tenderness to palpation is a sign of endomyometritis. Immediate treatment with broad spectrum antibiotics is recommended. Obtaining a sample from the endocervix for culture and sensitivity may be considered.

Delayed complications due to thermal damage to adjacent organs, such as the bladder and the bowel, may not become apparent until several weeks after surgery. A second postoperative visit is, therefore, scheduled within six weeks after surgery. The timing is individually assessed. The symptoms looked for are those of peritonitis, localized or generalized.

Further visits are planned at approximately 3 to 4 months after surgery and then on an annual basis. During this time, the cervical canal can be evaluated for patency.

The issue of fertility is discussed at these visits, especially if the patient presents with a regular menogram within 3 months after the procedure and no other method of sterilization has been performed.

RESULTS

Results can be looked at in two different ways. One can define success as no further need for treatment of the menorrhagia. The great majority of patients could then be considered "cured." If amenorrhea is considered the end point of the procedure, then one could say that the results are rather poor, since possibly as low as one-third of the patients will remain amenorrheic more than one year after surgery.

From August 1989 until June 1991, 90 patients underwent electrodesiccation of the endometrium using the roller ball technique described earlier. Table 11-1 shows the author's results plus those found in the literature. These results were obtained after at least 2 years of follow-up. The category "amenorrhea" has been intentionally omitted because of the difficulty in discerning minimal spotting from complete amenorrhea, both from the patient's and physician's point of view. Overall, 84.4% of the author's patients have less than two days of menstrual bleeding per month (average). These patients are satisfied with the result of the procedure. One patient underwent a hysterectomy because of persistent menorrhagia approximately three months after the ablation. Another underwent hysterectomy for persisting dysmenorrhea probably due to adenomyosis.

When comparing results published in the literature (4) (Table 11-3), the rates of success and failure appear to be independent of the method of ablation used.

The incidence of persisting dysmenorrhea, unfortunately, has not systematically been recorded in this series of patients. Meanwhile, it is recognized that persisting and de novo dysmenorrhea are problems requiring our attention. In my experience, dysmenorrhea has been a reason for further surgical treatment in only a few patients. However, it has spurred more caution in selecting candidates for the procedure.

The impact of electrodesiccation of the endometrium on premenstrual symptoms (PMS) is a subject of heated debate. One fallacy of this discussion is that patients undergoing endometrial ablation, who happen to have PMS, also have excessive bleeding. In addition, the clinical entity "PMS" is ill-defined, to say the least. Notwithstanding the above, empirical observations confirm that reducing the bulk of the endometrial tissue has more consequences than simple reduction of menstrual flow.

TABLE 11-3

Results

	N	HYPOMENORRHEA	EUMENORRHEA	FAILED
Author	90	76 (84.4%)	11 (12.2%)	3 (3.3%)
Nd-YAG	1560	983 (85%)	83 (5.3%)	102 (7%)
Resectoscope	786	534 (80%)	51 (8%)	85 (13%)
Combined	200	166 (97%)	1 (0.5%)	4 (2.5%)

Lefler and colleagues (2) performed interesting studies evaluating the impact of endometrial ablation on PMS symptoms. There was a statistically significant reduction in the severity of symptoms after endometrial ablation. This reduction persisted for at least three months. Studies with follow-up longer than one year are, as of yet, unpublished. Although these beneficial side effects of endometrial ablation are welcomed by the patients, it should be emphasized that PMS is not an indication to perform endometrial ablation. The main reason for this cautionary statement is that the currently available data have been obtained in women with menorrhagia as the primary complaint. It is unknown whether women with normal menogram would benefit in a similar fashion. The difficulty of defining "abnormal uterine bleeding" in objective numbers will certainly add to the confusion in designing and interpreting results of studies performed on women with apparently normal menses complaining of PMS symptoms.

CONCURRENT PROCEDURES

Laparoscopy is indicated in patients in whom pelvic pathology, such as endometriosis, is suspected. This is especially valuable if the patient is complaining of pelvic pain with or without dysmenorrhea. The presence of endometriosis is not a contraindication to endometrial ablation. If pelvic pain is a major complaint of the patient besides heavy menstrual bleeding, it is recommended to evaluate the pain with care because the persistence of pain may represent a serious challenge in the further management of the patient.

Laparoscopy to monitor the procedure is not recommended because this additional procedure will not prevent the occurrence of complications, such as perforation. The objective of a laparoscopy is to assess the damage that was caused by such a complication. This surgical management decision can be taken at the time of occurrence. Systematic scheduling of laparoscopy is not warranted.

REFERENCES

1. Bardenheuer, FH. Elektrokoagulation der Uterusschleimhaut zur Behandlung klimakterischer Blutungen. Zentralblatt Gynaekologie 1937; 59:209–216.
2. Lefler HT, Lefler CF. Improvement in PMS related to decrease in bleeding. J Reprod Med 1992;37:596–598.
3. Rose BD. Renal function and disorders of water and sodium balance. In: Rubenstein E, Federman D, eds. Medicine. New York: Scientific American, 1994;10(1):9–13.
4. Loffer F. Endometrial ablation—where do we stand? Gynecol Endosc 1992;1:175–179.
5. Whitelaw NL, Ewen SP, Pooley A, Haines P, Sutton CJG. Is there a role for contraception advice following endometrial ablation? Gynecol Endosc 1994 (in press).
6. Goldrath MH. Use of danazol in hysteroscopic surgery for menorrhagia. J Reprod Med 1990;35:91–96.

12

Control of Menorrhagia by Endometrial Resection

Adam Magos

A BRIEF HISTORY OF ENDOMETRIAL RESECTION

It is somewhat surprising that the first hysteroscopic endometrial ablations were performed using laser energy rather than electrosurgery, bearing in mind the relatively short history of the former and the long one of the latter in the field of medicine. Nonetheless, the original series of Nd–YAG laser ablations published by Goldrath in 1981 (1) was only followed two years later by a report from DeCherney's group at Yale, in the USA, when for the first time they used the resectoscope to control intractable uterine hemorrhage by electrocautery of the endometrium (2). Neuwirth, who pioneered hysteroscopic resection of submucous fibroids as far back as 1978 (3), also wrote about the possibility for the treatment of menorrhagia by resecting the endometrium in 1983, but did not include any cases in his review article (4). Indeed, the second ever paper in the English-speaking literature was also from Yale; in 1987, DeCherney and colleagues wrote an update of their earlier work and first referred to actual resection of the endometrium, rather than solely cautery, in a total of 21 patients (5). In contrast, by 1987, there were already five published series of laser ablations involving over 300 patients, by authors such as Goldrath, Daniel, Lomano, and Loffer, with many more publications to come in the ensuing few years.

The initial developments in the use of the resectoscope as a means of treating menorrhagia as an alternative to hysterectomy used instrumentation that, in general, consisted of a single-flow urological resectoscope combined with dextran 70 (Hyskon) as the uterine distention medium. The next phase of evolution of the technique of endometrial resection as well as wider application of this mode of treatment for the management of dysfunctional uterine bleeding involved two important modifications of the procedures described by DeCherney (2,5). First, electrolyte-free, low-viscosity fluids were used for uterine distention in place of dextran 70, thus allowing uterine irrigation as well as distention during surgery. Second, a continuous flow resectoscope for intrauterine surgery was designed, and this instrument was used to perform hysteroscopic myomectomy (6). The combination of nonviscous irrigant with a continuous flow sheathing system meant that the operative environment could be easily controlled to produce optimum conditions for safe intrauterine surgery. From this was born the treatment Hamou described as "partial endometrial resection," which involved the excision of the endometrium and the underlying 2 to 3 mm of myometrium over the upper uterine cavity. He used sterile 1.5% glycine solution as the distention medium and a standard 26 French continuous-flow urological resectoscope fitted with a 4-mm 30° foroblique telescope (in contrast to the Hallez myoma resectoscope, which only measured 21 French in diameter and utilized a 2.7-mm 0° endoscope).

With minor modifications, Hamou's instrumentation and technique have become the standard for endometrial resection as practiced by most gynecologists today. Two further developments have been the resection of the entire endometrial surface down to the upper endocervical canal (total transcervical resection of the endometrium [TCRE]) (7,8), and performing surgery under local rather than general anesthesia as an outpatient procedure (9,10).

Not unexpectedly, a procedure that offered a genuine alternative to hysterectomy with advantages in terms of lower cost, shorter operating time, reduced hospitalization, and faster recovery was quickly seized upon by both the public and gynecologists. Within two years of its introduction into the UK, for instance, almost half the acute hospitals were offering endometrial resection as a treatment for menorrhagia, in contrast to under 10% who were performing laser ablation (11). Although the results of longer follow-up studies and controlled comparisons with hysterectomy are only now becoming available, endometrial resection has already made a deep inroad into routine gynecological practice worldwide for one of the most common of gynecological disorders.

INDICATIONS AND CONTRAINDICATIONS

The truth is that endometrial ablation is still too much in its infancy for scientifically proven hard and fast rules about indications and contraindications. Nonetheless, the gradual publication of larger series of cases with longer follow-up periods has meant that patterns of success and failure are beginning to emerge, which serve as useful guides to patients and clinicians. The criteria developed in our clinic over the years (Table 12-1) are based on the observations that TCRE: (1) is a surgical procedure with potential complications, (2) does not predictably induce amenorrhea, (3) is less successful when there is gross pelvic pathology, (4) inhibits or adversely affects future pregnancies, and (5) is too new for us to know its long-term consequences.

The first matter to establish when assessing a potentially suitable patient is the severity of her symptoms. This is more difficult than might be thought as the menstrual history is a relatively poor indicator of genuine menorrhagia as judged by menstrual blood loss studies (12). Unfortunately, objective measurement of menstrual bleeding is not widely available in ordinary clinic practice, but daily pictorial charting of menstruation has been shown to be a reasonable

TABLE 12-1

Criteria for endometrial resection of the Minimally Invasive Therapy Unit and Endoscopy Training Center

INDICATIONS	CONTRAINDICATIONS
Menstrual problems justifying hysterectomy	Mild menstrual symptoms
Symptoms resistant to medical therapy	Not tried medical therapy
No desire for further pregnancies	Wish for further pregnancies
Regular, relatively short heavy periods	Irregular, prolonged periods
Satisfied with reduction in menstrual flow	Wants amenorrhea
No other significant problems indicating a need for a hysterectomy	Other significant problems indicating a need for a hysterectomy, (e.g., uterovaginal prolapse, congestive dysmenorrhea, chronic pelvic inflammatory disease, endometriosis, pelvic mass, cervical atypia)
Benign endometrial histology	Malignant or premalignant endometrial histology, e.g., atypical hyperplasia
Uterine size smaller than the equivalent of 12-week pregnancy (or uterine cavity length < 10 cm)	Large uterus greater than the equivalent of 12-week pregnancy (or uterine cavity length > 10 cm)
Submucous fibroids < 5 cm in diameter	Submucous fibroids > 5 cm diameter
Careful counseling, e.g., nature of treatment, recovery, likely menstrual result, fertility implications, unknown long-term consequences	Not able to be counseled adequately, e.g., communication or language problems

alternative and should be more widely administered (13). Women found to have menstrual blood loss within normal limits respond well to reassurance, explanation, and counselling, and often require no further treatment (14).

The second decision that has to be made is whether surgery or medical treatment should be tried in the first instance. Our current view is that TCRE is an alternative to hysterectomy rather than to nonsurgical treatment, with the implication that conservative pharmacological therapy should always be the first choice, and surgery should only be offered if this proves unsuccessful or is not tolerated because of side effects. The same considerations apply to women wishing to retain their fertility and for whom medical therapy is suitable.

Once it has been established that surgery is indicated, the menstrual pattern should be recorded because it is important to distinguish women with regular heavy periods from those with irregular, prolonged bleeding episodes; as none of the ablation techniques can guarantee amenorrhea, the latter patients may well remain dissatisfied because of their continued abnormal timing and duration, even if their menses become considerably lighter following surgery. The possible exception to this rule is if discrete intrauterine lesions (e.g., polyps, submucous fibroids) are found preoperatively whose simultaneous removal may regulate and shorten menstruation.

This leads to the important point of patient expectations regarding endometrial ablations. There are a minority of women who want a complete end to their menstrual cycle and for whom nothing less than amenorrhea will offer a "cure from the curse." These women are not good candidates for TCRE or any other ablative techniques for the reasons already given, and for them, hysterectomy, preferably by the vaginal route, is the ideal and only guaranteed solution. Hysterectomy also may well be indicated in the presence of obvious pelvic pathology, such as uterovaginal prolapse or pelvic mass, in women affected by severe premenstrual, congestive-type dysmenorrhea suggestive of endometriosis or chronic pelvic inflammatory disease and in those with a history of cervical dysplasia. TCRE per se will obviously not help any of these conditions, and the logical management is more radical surgery. The suggestion that endometrial ablation improves premenstrual tension, a condition characterized by multiple symptoms and almost certainly multiple pathophysiology, remains to be confirmed by larger studies (15).

The rationale of hysterectomy must be applied even more strictly to women found on biopsy to have endometrial malignancy or atypia. There can be no doubt that frank endometrial carcinoma should be treated in part by hysterectomy. Equally, atypical hyperplasia of the endometrium should also be managed similarly for the simple reason that the endometrium is rarely, if ever, excised completely, and therefore, it is not possible to guarantee against persistent recurrence of the endometrial abnormality. Simple, nonatypical hyperplasia is not thought to be premalignant, and therefore can be managed in menorrhagic women by ablation (16).

Once it has been decided that, in principle at least, TCRE is an appropriate mode of management for a particular patient, then the practicalities of the procedure should be considered based in the main on careful clinical examination supplemented by special investigations in some. Above all, account has to be taken of uterine size, as surgery becomes progressively more difficult, more time-consuming, and more hazardous with increasing size of the uterine cavity. Enlarged uteri are generally associated with the presence of myoma, and relatively large fibroids—relative, that is, to the size of the instruments used for TCRE—are difficult to excise completely hysteroscopically. Therefore, we tend to adhere to the limits of uterine and fibroid size listed in Table 12-1. Although these are only guidelines and women with uteri outside these limits have been treated, there seems to be little doubt that surgery is often complicated in these cases by fluid absorption and incomplete resection, leading ultimately to failure to relieve symptoms. Even with conservative estimates, it has nonetheless been judged that almost 60% of women with menorrhagia who currently undergo hysterectomy could be treated by TCRE (17).

The final component of the assessment process is as important as the rest and involves careful counselling of the patient so she understands fully the nature of her treatment and the likely menstrual outcome. Many of these aspects have already been touched upon. It should also be emphasized that TCRE is a relatively new procedure with no data regarding long-term follow-up, and, as such, there is no information regarding possible adverse sequelae, such as endometrial carcinoma. The policy in our hospital is to discuss this potential risk specifically, noting, however, that the chance of this complication developing in years to come may, in fact, be reduced by procedures such as TCRE simply because most of the endometrium is removed during the surgery. We openly admit that we do not as yet know the malignant risk of the procedure.

PREOPERATIVE ASSESSMENT

Apart from the routine checks of the patient's blood count and blood group, cervical smear, and, possibly, investigation of hormone and clotting status, pelvic ultrasound, diagnostic hysteroscopy, and endometrial biopsy are useful investigations before surgery to ensure that nothing unexpected will be found at the time of surgery. These additional investigations are complementary and especially indicated in women over the age of 45 years, and at any age in those with an enlarged uterus or adnexal mass, or if there is coexisting menstrual irregularity characterized by prolonged or irregular periods or intermenstrual or postcoital bleeding.

Scan of the pelvis will not only delineate any uterine fibroids and give their size but may suggest the presence of endometrial polyps or show an ovarian cyst. Diagnostic hysteroscopy and target biopsy are the optimum investigation for detecting small intrauterine lesions and the best technique for assessing the position and number of submucous fibroids and for deciding on their "resectability." Briefly, small myomas predominantly in the uterine cavity are the most suitable for simultaneous resection, while large ones deeply embedded in the myometrium are likely to be impossible to excise completely. If submucous fibroids are found, hysteroscopic myomectomy alone should be considered as an alternative mode of management to endometrial ablation. While myomectomy cannot offer the chance of amenorrhea, the menstrual benefits can still be considerable with the added advantage of leaving the uterine cavity intact (18). Conversely, the presence of relatively large intramural fibroids, impossible to treat concurrently but that nonetheless will tend to make the resection more difficult, should act as a warning and either rollerball coagulation (19), laser ablation with possible myolysis (20), or even hysterectomy should be offered to such patients.

Dilatation and curettage (D & C) is no longer indicated either as a diagnostic check or therapeutic intervention in menorrhagic patients. It is not as sensitive or specific as hysteroscopy in terms of detecting intrauterine lesions (21), and its beneficial effect on menstrual blood loss is short-lived, generally no more than 1 to 2 cycles (22). Apart from these considerations, it makes sense to assess a patient due to undergo a procedure involving operative hysteroscopy by the same modality, namely diagnostic hysteroscopy.

ENDOMETRIAL PREPARATION

The aim of all forms of endometrial ablation is to destroy or excise the full thickness of the endometrium. So, it seems logical to assume that preoperative preparation of the patient with the aim of thinning the endometrium to 1 to 2 mm would facilitate surgery (23) (see Chapter 7). Unfortunately, prospective randomized studies addressing this issue have yet to be published, so it is impossible to make recommendations based on scientific fact. Certainly, most reports of laser endometrial ablation include pretreatment with agents, such as danazol or a GnRH analog as a means of ensuring a sufficiently thin endometrium for full-thickness coagulation or vaporization, the tissue effect typically being 4 to 5 mm (24). As the tissue results of rollerball coagulation are similar to laser, the initial studies of rollerball ablation also utilized pretreatment, not only with the above agents but also progestogens and the combined contraceptive pill (19,25). More recently, curettage of the endometrium immediately prior to rollerball ablation has been suggested as an alternative to pharmacological preparation, with advantages in terms of reduced treatment costs and avoidance of side effects, which can make pretreatment intolerable (26). The simple measure of operating in the immediate postmenstrual phase of the cycle is another means of ensuring a relatively thin endometrium in most patients, but this is logistically a difficult task in health care systems with long waiting lists for surgery.

Endometrial thickness is not so critical with endometrial resection, where the tissue is excised rather than coagulated, and resection can continue until the myometrial fibers are visualized. This could mean that several cuts have to be made in each area to excise and, indeed, undercut the basal endometrium by 2 to 3 mm, bearing in mind that the cutting loop used by most hysteroscopists has a diameter of 8 mm with a cutting depth of 4 to 5 mm. Thus, treatment of a patient who has thick, premenstrual endometrium will take longer, and this will be associated with a greater risk of complications, such as fluid overload, which is, to some extent, time-dependent. There are other disadvantages to this scenario. Visualization of the uterine cavity is more difficult when the endometrium is lush and the risk of accidental uterine perforation theoretically greater, particularly in the ostial areas, where the myometrium is normally relatively thin. The fluffy nature of untreated endometrium tends to cause obstruction to the small outflow holes of the resectoscope sheath, thereby disturbing the dynamics of uterine distention/irrigation with not only a deterioration of the endoscopic view but a tendency for an increase in intrauterine pressure, and, thus, in the rate of fluid absorption (27). Whether endometrial preparation with GnRH analogs has an additional benefit on fluid absorption as a result of changes in uterine and endometrial vasculature remains to be seen (28).

Whatever the ultimate advantages and disadvantages of preoperative endometrial thinning, there can be little doubt that endometrial resection is easier to perform in women who have been prepared, and this is to be highly recommended for the resectionist-in-training.

ANTIBIOTICS

As with endometrial preparation, no firm recommendations can be given regarding the use of prophylactic antibiotics during surgery. In some respects, hysteroscopic surgery is comparable to vaginal surgery, where antibiotics are widely used at hysterectomy. Although the vaginal vault is not opened as at hysterectomy, about 20% of the uterine irrigant absorbed during surgery escapes into the peritoneal cavity via the fallopian tubes (29). Of even more concern is that the remaining 80% enters the circulation directly via the myometrial vasculature, and, although the distention media used are sterile preparations, they are not intended for intravenous use. For all these reasons, we do give our patients prophylactic antibiotics as a single dose, currently a combination of metronidazole (1 gram per rectum one hour before surgery) and a third-generation cephalosporin (cefotaxime 750 mg IV at the time of surgery).

TYPE OF RESECTOSCOPE

Resectoscopic instrumentation has already been discussed in detail in Chapter 2. Resectoscopes used for hysteroscopic surgery share a common origin in the form of the urological resectoscope, and there is little difference between the various manufacturers' designs. Nonetheless, there are various combinations of size, sheathing system, handle mechanism, and optic available, and our current choice is described in Table 12-2. As can be seen, we favor a medium-sized instrument fitted with an angled endoscope. As we use a nonviscous distention medium (1.5% glycine solution), a continuous flow system with inflow and outflow sheaths is ideal for easy control of uterine distention and irrigation. Most importantly, from a safety aspect, we favor a passive type of handle mechanism, whereby the cutting loop sits protected inside the inflow sheath at rest and is only pushed out immediately prior to a cut being made. This arrange-

TABLE 12-2

Basic Equipment and Settings for Endometrial Resection

1. Resectoscope	26 French gauge continuous flow sheath
	24 French cutting loop
	Passive handle mechanism
	4-mm 30° foroblique telescope
2. Irrigation system	Sterile 1.5% glycine solution
	Hamou hysteromat set at:
	100 to 125 mmHg irrigation pressure
	50 mmHg suction pressure
	300 mL/min maximum flow rate
3. Electrosurgical generator	e.g., Valleylab Force 2 set at:
	100 to 125 watts cutting power
	Blend 1 to 3
	50 W coagulating power
4. Illumination and video	High intensity cold light source (at least 250 W)
	Wide light cable
	Video camera
	High resolution color monitor

ment makes accidental trauma to the uterus unlikely as inadvertent activation of the electrode cannot have any tissue effect under normal circumstances.

Almost as important as the characteristics of the resectoscope itself is the coupling of the optic to a high-resolution color monitor via a small-chip video camera. The advantages are considerable in terms of operator comfort, particularly with patients with an acutely anteverted uterus, in whom the non-video alternative would be to operate kneeling on the floor, and for the teaching and supervision of beginners. An indirect benefit is the possibility for patients who have their surgery under local or regional anesthesia to watch their procedure, something which a surprisingly large proportion of our patients opt for in fact (8).

IRRIGATION SYSTEM

A discussion about irrigation fluids and systems used for hysteroscopic surgery has been given in Chapter 5. Briefly, the first hysteroscopic myomectomies and endometrial ablations were carried out using dextran 70 as the distention medium, but most ablations are now performed using isotonic (or near isotonic) low-viscosity fluids, such as normal saline or Ringer's lactate, if using laser, and 1.5% glycine or 3% or 5% sorbitol for electrosurgical procedures, such as TCRE. As only electrolyte-free solutions can be used with electrosurgery, absorption of these fluids can be associated with the development of electrolyte disturbances, of which hyponatremia is clinically the most important.

The uterine cavity, being a potential space, has to be distended under pressure to allow for an adequate panoramic view for surgery. In practice, this means a clear view of the uterine fundus. Uterine compliance seems to be highly variable, perhaps influenced by uterine size, the presence of fibroids, and endometrial thickness, but typically, pressures of 80 to 100 mmHg have to be reached for adequate distention of the cavity. Uterine distention of this magnitude can be achieved in a number of ways, including gravity feed systems or with dedicated pumps. When faced with problems of insufficient distention or a cloudy view, it is important to realize that it is the irrigation pressure that controls the former and the suction pressure that regulates the latter under normal circumstances.

Whatever distention/irrigation system is used for TCRE, it is essential to monitor fluid balance throughout the procedure to avoid fluid overload by the simple measure of stopping surgery before dangerous volumes are absorbed. This is even more important with TCRE than with other ablative techniques for two reasons. First, electrolyte-free solutions are used for uterine distention with the risk of hyponatremia, which is proportional to the volume of fluid absorbed (29). Second, as surgery involves resecting across blood vessels, intravasation of the irrigant is more likely than with rollerball or laser ablation, where the endometrium is coagulated.

ELECTROSURGICAL GENERATOR

The resectoscope is an electrosurgical instrument that uses monopolar current for its tissue effect of cutting or coagulation. It is important for the surgeon to understand the theory of electrosurgery outlined in Chapters 3 and 4. Modern solid-state electrosurgical generators should be used as these tend to have an increasing number of safety features built into them and provide accurate control of power output. Two principles must be remembered to minimize the risk of electrosurgical burns to patients: there must be no malfunction or break in the electrical circuit, and the lowest power setting should be used that produces the desired tissue effect. The latter will vary depending on the make and model of the generator and resectoscope, so it is only possible to give approximate guidelines as to the power settings (Table 12-2). Basically, the uterine tissue should cut with ease, with little or no drag on the cutting loop during resection. This can be achieved by using a pure cutting current, but we prefer to utilize a blended current to (1) provide additional hemostasis, (2) possibly reduce the volume of fluid absorbed by intravasation as a result, and (3) increase the depth of thermal damage to the underlying myometrium and, thereby, at least in theory, lead to coagulation of any unresected islands of endometrium (30,31). The penalties for operating with a mixed cutting/coagulating current are that higher powers have to be employed, there is a tendency for charring of the tissues, which may make identification of the myometrial fibers more difficult, and the resected chips are more likely to stick to the cutting loop.

ANESTHESIA

Either general or regional anesthetic techniques can be used for endometrial resection (32). Endometrial ablation is not only a day-case procedure but one that can be performed using local anesthesia, intravenous sedation (or more correctly "anxiolysis"), and supplementary intravenous analgesia, a combination that has advantages in terms of medical manpower, turnaround time, and patient recovery (9,32). Local anesthesia is sufficient because the sensory nerve supply to the uterus is relatively insensitive to noxious stimuli, such as cutting and heating, two of the modalities used in resection, although it is more sensitive to distention. This fact, combined with the well-known efficacy of what is often referred to as "sedoanalgesia" (sedation with analgesia) in many other branches of medicine for endoscopic and other invasive procedures, led us to develop this approach to the operation.

Briefly, patients now receive a premedication cocktail of temazepam 20 mg PO for sedation and a rectal suppository of diclofenac, 100 mg one hour before surgery. In the anesthetic room (or operating theatre or endoscopy suite), baseline readings of heart rate, electrocardiogram, oxygen saturation, and blood pressure are taken, to be continued during surgery. A small intravenous dose of an opiate analgesic, e.g., fentanyl 50 μg) is then given, followed 5 minutes later by an anxiolytic, e.g., midazolam 2.5 mg; the dose of the anxiolytic is subsequently titrated in 1 mg increments until the patient is relaxed (but not asleep). We routinely give facial oxygen, as both fentanyl and midazolam are potent respiratory depressants.

When comfortable and relaxed, the patient is placed in lithotomy position and prepared for surgery in the usual manner. The cervix is grasped with a tenaculum and 10 mL of 1% lignocaine containing 1:200,000 adrenaline is injected into the paracervical nerve plexus (2.5 mL at 3, 5, 7, and 9 o'clock behind the cervix, respectively) and a similar volume into the substance of the cervix. While the local anaesthetic takes effect, the resectoscope is assembled with an injection cannula rather than a cutting electrode and connected to the irrigation system, electrosurgical generator, light source, and video camera ready for surgery. The position of the patient, surgeon, and equipment is shown in Figure 12-1.

By the time the anesthetic has taken effect, the uterine cavity can be sounded and the cervix dilated without discomfort to the

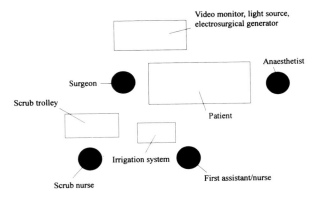

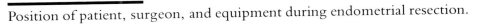

FIGURE 12-1

Position of patient, surgeon, and equipment during endometrial resection.

patient. The resectoscope is then introduced into the uterine cavity and a further 20 mL of the lignocaine/adrenaline mixture is injected at 10 to 15 points into the myometrium to a depth of 1 cm. Most of the injections are made around the uterine fundus and cornua, the areas the least anesthetized by the paracervical block. Surgery can then commence as under general anesthesia, additional small doses of fentanyl or midazolam being administered if further analgesia or axiolysis is required; on average, 75 to 100 μg of fentanyl together with 5 to 7.5 mg of midazolam is ultimately given.

The choice of anesthesia must be dictated by the patient's comfort and tolerance of the procedure. However, there are high-risk patients who are unsuitable for general anesthesia for whom TCRE under local anesthesia offers the chance of surgery (10). Conversely, it must not be thought that surgery under local anesthesia and sedation is an "office" procedure. There has to be a dedicated member of the medical staff, not necessarily an anesthetist, who is responsible for sedation and monitoring of the patient. Close and continuous monitoring of respiratory function and other vital signs is mandatory, and facilities for resuscitation, intubation, and of course laparotomy, have to be available. Lastly, the operator should be someone experienced, who can complete the required surgery quickly, efficiently, and safely.

SURGICAL TECHNIQUE

There are many similarities between TCRE and the other hysteroscopic techniques of endometrial ablation. The patient is positioned and prepared as for a dilatation and curettage, and there is no need to catheterize the bladder unless it is full and making uterine palpation difficult. The operating table is tilted slightly head-down to encourage the bowel to fall away from the uterus and, thereby, make bowel trauma less likely should the uterus be perforated during surgery. There is a danger of air embolization in this position should air enter the uterine irrigation circuit (34), but this is unlikely, particularly when gravity is used to pressurize the uterus. As an alternative safety measure, introducing a hydroperitoneum to float the bowel off the uterus has been suggested, but this seems unnecessarily invasive for a risk so slight.

The uterus is examined bimanually, the cavity sounded, and the cervix dilated to admit the resectoscope easily but prevent leakage around the outflow sheath. For instance, if using a 26 French gauge resectoscope, which has an outer diameter of just under 9 mm, dilatation to Hegar 10 is adequate and will ensure that loss of irrigant between the sheath and the cervix is minimal. The resectoscope is then introduced into the endocervical canal, the irrigation system opened, and the instrument guided into the uterine cavity under direct vision rather than blindly by means of an obturator.

After inspection of the cavity and injection of local anesthesia if required, the resection begins systematically in the following order: the uterine fundus and ostial areas, the upper half of the cavity starting posteriorly and working around either clockwise or counterclockwise, a similar sequence in the lower half of the cavity, and finally, resection of the top half of the endocervical canal in women undergoing total TCRE (35). The fundus is treated first as it is the most difficult area to resect with the greatest risk of uterine perforation in the thin ostial regions and the part of the uterus that becomes obscured most quickly by the resected chippings. Similarly, as the endometrial pieces tend to sink to the bottom of the uterine cavity, it is best to resect the posterior wall early on when treating the body of the uterus.

As it is mechanically difficult to resect the fundal endometrium with a standard backward-angled or right-angled cutting loop, a forward-angled electrode is used for this part of the procedure. It is a conventional cutting loop bent forward manually to 10° to 15° off the perpendicular (Figure 12-2). Rather than bending the loops backward and forward during surgery, a few loops are kept at the desired angle for resecting the fundus and cornual areas and changed for the standard backward-angled loop when the remainder of the cavity is to be treated. Even with this precaution, the endometrium has to be undercut between the two cornua in a series of small chips, taking care not to push the loop more deeply into the myometrium than is necessary. Particular care has to be taken over the two tubal ostia, where the myometrium is at its thinnest, and it is best to take a series of shallow shavings until all the endometrium has been resected here rather than make one large cut and risk perforation. Alternatively, the fundus and cornual regions can be coagulated using a rollerball before switching to loop-resection for the rest of the procedure (36).

After the fundus, the rollerball or forward-angled loop is changed for a standard backward-angled loop that rests inside the

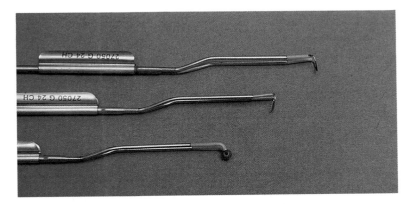

FIGURE 12-2

Cutting loops used for resecting the uterine fundus (top), rest of the cavity (middle), and rollerball (bottom).

insulated tip of the instrument (Figure 12-2). As this electrode does not protrude from the end of the irrigation sheaths, it is both safer and more efficient at cutting and should, therefore, be used as early as possible in the procedure. Rather than withdrawing the whole instrument from the uterus, it is easier to unlock the handle mechanism from the inflow sheath and merely remove this part of the resectoscope to change the electrode; it can then be reinserted directly into the uterine cavity via the sheathing system.

As gravity makes the resected tissue fall on to the posterior uterine wall, it makes sense to treat this part of the cavity first before it becomes obscured. Typically therefore, surgery is started laterally by one of the tubal ostia and continued over the posterior wall to the contralateral side and then on to the anterior wall in a circular fashion, the upper cavity being treated before the lower part of the uterus. The chips of tissue, typically measuring $2.5 \times 0.7 \times 0.5$ cm as a reflection of the travel of the handle mechanism and the size of the cutting loop, are herded towards the uterine fundus with the loop, leaving the cavity relatively clear for surgery. In this way, the resection can continue uninterrupted until the whole cavity has been treated, at which stage the pieces are removed with a flushing curette or similar instrument (Figures 12-3 through 12-5).

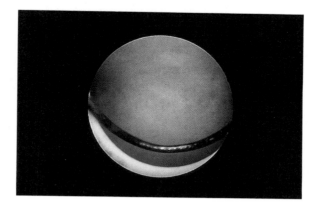

FIGURE 12-3

The appearance of the uterine cavity at the start of endometrial resection.

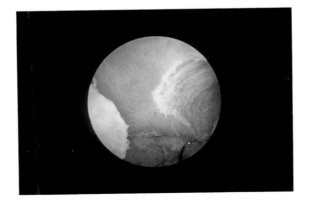

FIGURE 12-4

The endometrial/myometrial interface during surgery.

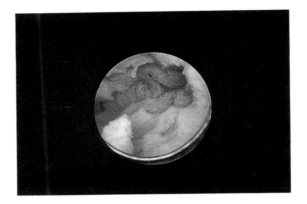

FIGURE 12-5

The appearance of the uterine cavity at the end of endometrial resection.

An alternative technique is to cut full-length chips from the fundus toward the uterine isthmus by moving the whole instrument while cutting before finally pulling in the handle mechanism to disconnect the tissue from the uterus. The resected piece is then generally removed from the cavity immediately as the view would become obscured relatively quickly by these larger chips. We do not favor this approach in all cases as it seems a less efficient method of operating from the point of view of speed, fluid leakage via the cervix, and the fact that each inflation/deflation cycle is associated with uterine bleeding, which further obscures the hysteroscopic view. However, we do use this technique when the endometrium is very thick, during repeat resections, and for removing larger submucous fibroids.

Whichever technique is used, the aim of surgery is to excise all the endometrium together with the underlying 2 to 3 mm of myometrium, which is sufficient to remove all but the deepest extensions of the endometrium but not too deep to cut into the larger branches of the uterine artery. The circular myometrial fibers are easily visualized during resection and, once reached, should only be resected further with great care as this may result in uterine perforation. If the endometrium has been prepared with an agent, such as danazol or a GnRH analog, it is unusual to need more than one cut to achieve the desired depth of resection.

The lower margin of resection can be just above the uterine isthmus (*partial resection*) or into the upper part of the endocervical canal (*total resection*). Total TCRE offers the only chance of amenorrhea, although as with any of the ablative techniques, this endpoint cannot be guaranteed. Nonetheless, most women opt for total rather than partial resection, which is performed by resecting superficially into the cervical substance. Severe cervical hemorrhage necessitating hysterectomy has been recorded (38), but we have not had such a complication in more than 600 procedures. As an alternative to resecting the upper endocervical canal, the rollerball can be used to ablate this area (36), although it could be argued that deep thermal damage and subsequent sloughing of the tissue could result in secondary hemorrhage.

Many patients with menorrhagia have submucous fibroids, and these can be excised easily at the time of endometrial resection provided the myoma are not numerous, are primarily intracavity in position, and are less than 4 to 5 cm in maximum diameter. Deeper fibroids are best left and only resected superficially to remove the overlying endometrium as deep resection would promote fluid absorption and hemorrhage and risk uterine perforation. It is doubtful if menorrhagic women with multiple deep fibroids are best treated by hysteroscopic surgery as opposed to hysterectomy.

At the end of surgery, once the uterus has been emptied of most of the endometrial/myometrial chips, the resectoscope is introduced back into the uterine cavity to check for any untreated areas or major bleeding points. The former are simply resected. This demonstrates the beauty of all visual techniques while the latter are coagulated using a loop or rollerball. Bleeding during surgery is usually minor because of the relatively high intrauterine pressure created by the irrigation system, but bleeding can be unmasked by lowering the distention pressure at the end of surgery. However, it is doubtful if it is worth spending time coagulating individual vessels or areas unless the hemorrhage is considerable.

All the collected resected tissue is sent for histological examination to exclude any unsuspected serious pathology. The availability of relatively intact tissue for such assessment is a major advantage of endometrial resection over other ablative techniques, which destroy the endometrium in situ, and endometrial carcinoma has been uncovered in this way despite previous normal endometrial assessment (16,37).

TIPS FOR EFFECTIVE USE OF THE RESECTOSCOPE

There are four basic principles that should be adhered to for effective resectoscopic surgery (Table 12-3). Firstly, it must be remembered that it is not the cutting loop that cuts the endometrium but the arc of the cutting current passing from it. The loop must, there-

TABLE 12-3

Tips for resecting effectively

1. It is the electrical current that cuts, not the loop.
2. Only cut when moving the loop towards the resectoscope sheath.
3. Continue cutting until the loop is totally within the sheath.
4. Apply sufficient pressure between the loop and uterus when cutting.

fore, be energized to make a cut, and indeed, the electrosurgical generator should be activated just before the loop comes in contact with the surface tissue to allow space for a spark of current to form (39). Secondly, cutting should only take place when moving the loop towards the resectoscope sheath as an active loop pushed away from the sheath can easily perforate the uterus. Thirdly, the loop should be brought fully into the inner sheath before the generator is turned off in order to make a clean cut; otherwise a part of the resected tissue will remain attached to the uterus. Finally, the mobility of the uterus is such that a considerable pressure has to be applied between the cutting loop and the uterus during resection to avoid skimming the surface and making too shallow a cut. This is achieved by progressively angling the whole instrument while the loop is being pulled in, the cervix acting as the fulcrum for this movement.

TECHNICAL PROBLEMS DURING SURGERY

The most commonly encountered difficulties during and after endometrial resection are listed in Table 12-4 with the likely causes and appropriate solutions. From the point of view of both safety and efficacy, it is essential that throughout surgery there is (1) clear view of the uterine cavity, (2) properly functioning resectoscope, and (3) careful monitoring of fluid balance and vital signs. If there is any concern about these aspects of the procedure, then surgery should cease immediately, to be continued only if the situation has been rectified. TCRE may be a minor procedure in terms of surgical time, external trauma, and recovery, but it is major surgery in terms of potential risks.

OPERATIVE COMPLICATIONS

The operative and postoperative risks of endometrial resection are listed in Table 12-5. Published data have shown that these complica-

TABLE 12-4

Technical Problems and Solutions During Endometrial Resection

PROBLEM	CAUSE	SOLUTION
1. Poor uterine distention	Low distention pressure	Increase distention pressure
	Uterine perforation	Stop and check abdomen
	Cervical incompetence	Cervical suture or tenacula around cervix
2. Slow clearance of debris/blood	Insufficient suction pressure	Increase suction pressure
	Blocked outflow hole in sheath	Clean sheath
3. Inefficient cutting	Cutting power too low	Increase cutting power or reduce blend
	Cutting loop not in sheath at rest	Gently bend loop into correct position
	Cutting loop broken	Replace cutting loop
4. Poor view of endometrium and uterine cavity	Poor uterine distention	See problem no. 1
	Slow clearance of debris/blood	See problem no. 2
	Resected chips restrict view	Remove chips before continuing with surgery
	Bubbles on the anterior wall	Increase suction pressure
	Fibroids	Hysteroscopic total or partial myomectomy
5. Rapid fluid absorption	Distention pressure too high	Reduce distention pressure
	Uterine perforation	Stop and check cavity
6. Bleeding during surgery	Low distention pressure	Increase distention pressure
	Insufficient coagulation during cutting	Increase coagulation blend
	Resection too deep	Coagulate vessel(s) and resect more shallowly
	Fibroids	Coagulate vessels around pseudocapsule
7. Hemorrhage after surgery	Resection too deep	Uterine tamponade with balloon catheter
	Infection	Antibiotics
	Resected debris in cavity	Evacuate and give antibiotics

TABLE 12-5

Potential Complications of Endometrial Resection

| | POSTOPERATIVE | |
INTRAOPERATIVE	SHORT-TERM	LONG-TERM
Uterine perforation	Infection	Recurrence of symptoms
Fluid overload	Hematometra	Pregnancy
Primary hemorrhage	Secondary hemorrhage	Uterine malignancy
Gas embolism	Cyclical pain	
	Treatment failure	

tions are unusual and that TCRE is a relatively safe procedure in experienced hands (40). For instance, the incidence of serious intraoperative complications, such as uterine perforation, has been estimated at between 0.8 to 4% (41,42), fluid overload at 0 to 3% (8,42), and hemorrhage at 0.4 to 5% (8,36). Larger surveys have reported equally low incidence of complications (11,43). For instance, a postal questionnaire sent out to members of the British Society for Gynaecological Endoscopy analyzed 4038 procedures, including 2796 (70%) endometrial resections, found uterine perforation occurred in 1.1% of cases, with major visceral damage in 0.2%, fluid overload in 0.4%, and hemorrhage in 0.2% (43). Results showed that uterine perforation and related complications were associated with inexperience, 33% of the cases taking place during the surgeon's first procedure and over half during the first five. Fatalities from fluid overload or hemorrhage or sepsis secondary to uterine perforation have also been reported from Europe and the USA, but, generally, only as isolated and unpublished case histories. The current literature, however, suggests that both the minor and major morbidity as well as mortality associated with endometrial resection are considerably less than would be expected from hysterectomy (44,45). It is also hoped, although it remains to be proven by continued audit, that hysteroscopic procedures, such as TCRE, will not be associated with the same long-term potential complications of hysterectomy, such as premature ovarian failure (46), heart disease (47), and gastrointestinal dysfunction (48).

Uterine perforation is undoubtedly a major hazard of TCRE, inherently more so than with rollerball coagulation or laser ablation. If uterine perforation occurs while using the active electrode, surgery must stop immediately and laparotomy or laparoscopy performed, depending on the experience of the operator. It is vital for the safety of the patient that serious vascular, gastrointestinal, or urinary trauma is realized at once and corrective surgery performed during the same anesthetic. Provided the resection is stopped as soon as the perforation has been made, major intra-abdominal trauma is very much the exception rather than the rule. It is when the warning signs of uterine deflation with rapid fluid absorption are ignored and surgery continued that the scene is set for disaster. Conversely, we have managed several women with uterine perforation endoscopically by confirming a lack of major abdominal trauma laparoscopically, suturing the perforation laparoscopically, and then continuing with the hysteroscopic procedure once the uterus has been made "water tight" (49).

The absorption of too much uterine irrigant is the second major potential operative complication of endometrial resection. It is difficult to compare techniques as several factors influence fluid absorption (27,50,51), but the risk does not seem to be consistently different to other hysteroscopic ablative procedures despite the fact that it is the only one that involves transection of myometrial vessels. It is probable that fluid absorption per unit time is greater with TCRE, but as the operative time is faster, the total volume of irrigant absorbed is not more. Apart from fluid load, it must be remembered that only electrolyte-free solutions can be used with electrosurgical procedures, such as endometrial resection. This means that major metabolic disturbances will accompany fluid overload, characterized by a dilutional effect on serum electrolytes, most importantly sodium (52–55). Although hyponatremia is defined as serum Na^+ less than 125 mmol/L, what constitutes a clinically dangerous concentration in the setting of hysteroscopic surgery in otherwise healthy, relatively young, and usually fit women remains to be determined. Several authors agree that surgery should stop if the volume of fluid absorbed exceeds 1.5 to 2 L. In our institution, a strict protocol is followed in these situations as outlined in Table 12-6. Although careful monitoring of fluid balance during surgery is paramount, labelling of the irrigant fluid with 1% ethanol has been shown to be a useful index of dilutional change (56).

Hemorrhage during or after surgery is unusual, and, indeed, the operative blood loss during TCRE has been shown to be only 10 to 20 mL when measured objectively (38). As noted earlier, nonfatal gas embolism has been reported during endometrial resection (34), but this is preventable by ensuring that air does not enter the irrigation circuit. The incidence of infection following surgery is un-

TABLE 12-6

Management of Fluid Overload During Endometrial Resection

VOLUME ABSORBED	RISK AND ACTION
<1 L	Major cardiovascular/respiratory or metabolic disturbances unlikely
	CONTINUE WITH SURGERY
1–2 L	Major cardiovascular/respiratory or metabolic disturbance possible
	Monitor vital signs closely
	Check serum electrolytes
	Treat with IV diuretic, e.g., 20 mg frusemide
	Catheterize bladder and monitor urine output
	COMPLETE SURGERY AS QUICKLY AS POSSIBLE
>2 L	Major cardiovascular/respiratory or metabolic disturbances likely
	Actions as above if not already carried out
	Observe for at least 12 to 24 hours
	STOP SURGERY

known as hospitalization is so short; certainly, very few women give a history suggestive of intrauterine infection with an offensive vaginal discharge or lower abdominal tenderness, so the risk of sepsis must be considered to be low.

POSTOPERATIVE MANAGEMENT

TCRE is day-case surgery in most cases and, potentially, an outpatient procedure if performed under local anesthesia. Pain is generally slight and adequately treated by nonopiate oral analgesics. Nausea is also uncommon unless there has been a degree of fluid overload (51). Bleeding tends to be heavy for the first 24 hours or so before gradually reducing over the next 1 to 3 weeks to be followed by a nonoffensive discharge for a short while (8). Antibiotics are rarely given after surgery unless the uterus has been perforated. Normal activities and work can be resumed soon after surgery. The variations in recovery seen in clinical practice are more a testament to the important influences of personality and culture rather than the trauma of the operation itself. Resumption of sexual intercourse is generally advised only after bleeding has stopped.

Women are now reviewed three months after surgery as it is difficult to judge the menstrual effects of TCRE before then. There is no published data regarding the use of postoperative endometrial suppression with agents such as danazol, long-acting progestogen injections, or GnRH analogs as there is with laser ablation and rollerball coagulation, but there is some evidence that at least the early amenorrhea rates can be considerably increased by such a maneuver (Shaxted E, personal communication).

RESULTS OF SURGERY

Data regarding the menstrual results of endometrial resection as opposed to the other ablative techniques, such as rollerball coagulation and especially Nd–YAG laser ablation, are not widely available. Distinction also has to be made between those series where the cutting loop of the resectoscope is used primarily as a coagulating tool, much like a rollerball, and where it is used to perform endometrial resection proper, the subject of this chapter. Thus, the original paper by DeCherney and Polan in 1983 (2), their larger follow-up series in 1987 (5), and the study by Derman and coworkers with an 8 year follow-up (57), all essentially describe the results of endometrial coagulation with the cutting loop rather than TCRE. Other series mix techniques, even to the extent of including endometrial resection, rollerball coagulation, and laser ablation on the same patients (58).

Experience regarding pure endometrial resection, with rollerball coagulation of the cornual and cervical regions in some cases, come mainly from Europe and Australia. These studies come broadly to the same conclusion, that the menstrual results of surgery are comparable to the other ablative procedures, with amenorrhea in about one-third of patients and failure in approximately one in six (7,8,36,40,41,59,60). Periods tend not only to become lighter but also shorter and less painful. Surgery can be effective when treating relatively enlarged uteri with simultaneous hysteroscopic myomectomy. TCRE has also been used effectively in atypical situations, such as after radiotherapy for cervical carcinoma (61). Menstrual blood loss studies have also confirmed that TCRE is followed by a significant reduction in bleeding, by an average of 77% after total resection, and 66% after partial resection (62,63).

How do these results compare with other methods of endometrial ablation? It is, in fact, almost impossible to make a proper comparison as so many variables influence the results of surgery. The experience of the surgeon, age of the patient, presence of uterine pathology, such as myomas, and the use of endometrial preparation and postoperative suppression are just a few of the factors that have to be allowed for. For instance, as the resectoscope was used initially to excise submucous fibroids, it is not surprising that women with even relatively large myomatous uteri tend to be offered hysteroscopic resection, whereas laser ablation is mainly reserved for those with dysfunctional bleeding.

An even more important consideration is the duration of follow-up of the study groups, as there is now good evidence that the rate of treatment failure, as to be expected, increases with time. We have recently analyzed our results using life table methods looking at finite endpoints, such as the need for repeat resection or hysterectomy (as opposed to endpoints such as satisfaction and amenorrhea, which can change over time and are thus not suitable for this type of analysis). As can be seen clearly from Figures 12-6 through 12-8, the chance of undergoing further treatment increases progressively over time, the rate depending to some extent on the nature of the initial procedure. For instance, there is a 19% chance of further surgery, including a 12% chance of hysterectomy, being performed within four years of a total (or intended total) TCRE, 30% and 9%, respectively, after partial TCRE, and 40% and 40%, respectively, after a repeat TCRE. This trend of gradual failure with time means that overall success rates based on patients who have recently undergone surgery as well as those treated some time ago will give a falsely optimistic picture

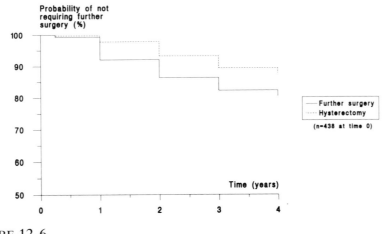

FIGURE 12-6

Life table analysis of the need for further surgery after intended total TCRE.

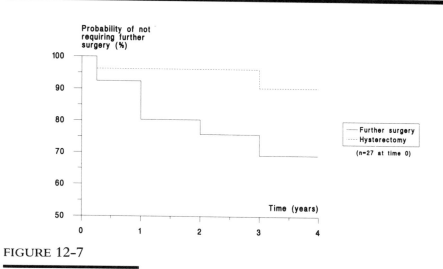

FIGURE 12-7

Life table analysis of the need for further surgery after partial TCRE.

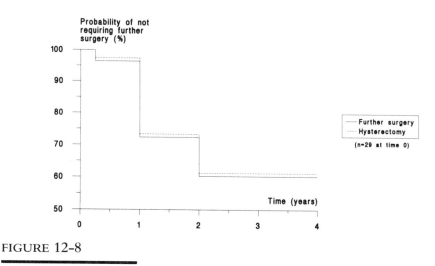

FIGURE 12-8

Life table analysis of the need for further surgery after repeat total TCRE.

regarding the success of the procedure, and yet, this is exactly the way that most authors present their results (24,40). Interestingly, one study reported that while the achievement of amenorrhea after TCRE is related to operator experience, the chance of treatment failure, at least in the short term, is not (64).

Control of Menorrhagia by Endometrial Resection   243

The importance of treatment failure is well demonstrated by controlled studies of TCRE versus hysterectomy. The two studies so far published, both from the UK, confirm all the expected benefits of the lesser procedure in terms of reduced operating time, shorter hospitalization, faster recovery, and cost savings (65,66). However, despite the relatively short follow-up periods in these studies, the need for further treatment, an index of patient satisfaction, and efficacy, were superior after hysterectomy. Preliminary analysis of our own multicenter study suggests a similar picture (Magos AL, unpublished data). The need for further treatment after endometrial ablation, of course, has important financial implications, and it may be that if a large enough proportion of women undergoing hysteroscopic surgery ultimately fail with their treatment, then hysterectomy may become a less expensive option overall (67).

LONG-TERM COMPLICATIONS

The postoperative complications of endometrial ablation are also listed in Table 12-5. Apart from treatment failure (or recurrence of symptoms some time after surgery), pelvic pain, hematometra, and pregnancy are most often seen. Although menstrual pain is usually helped by surgery, in contrast to premenstrual dsymenorrhea, a small proportion of women do develop cyclical pain that is worse than preoperatively or that arises de novo. In a certain number, the pain is related to the development of a hematometra secondary to a combination of residual endometrium in the uterine cavity and cervical stenosis, clue to the diagnosis being the absence of menstruation despite the pain (8,68). The collection is generally fundal and presumably linked to too shallow resection in the cornual areas for fear of uterine perforation. Treatment in these cases is relatively simple and involves cervical dilatation and drainage of the hematometra followed by a repeat ablation if amenorrhea is desired. Extra care has to be taken if resection is to be carried out as the myometrium has already been thinned once by the initial procedure, and rollerball coagulation would seem a safer option unless the uterine wall is known to be thick because of intramural fibroids.

More difficult to treat are those women whose pelvic pain is not associated with hematometra. Cases have been reported of granulomatous endometritis in this situation (69,70). Laparoscopy can be useful to detect pelvic pathology such as the presence of endometriosis. However, the laparoscopic exam often shows no abnormalities. In these cases, laparoscopic uterine nerve ablation or presacral neurectomy could be offered, but in our limited experience, the results of the former have been poor. Ultimately, most of these patients will request the final cure, hysterectomy, and in some cases, adenomyosis will be the ultimate diagnosis.

Endometrial resection should not be considered an absolute contraceptive, and there have been several reports in the literature of pregnancy after TCRE, both intrauterine and ectopic (71–73). While most women choose to undergo termination of pregnancy in this situation, those who continue appear to be at an increased risk of complications, such as prematurity, growth retardation, and the need for abdominal delivery. A rare fetal anomaly has also been reported affecting a pregnancy after endometrial ablation (single suture craniosynostosis), but it was felt that the two were not directly linked (72). For these reasons, women at risk of pregnancy after endometrial ablation should be offered effective sterilization or advised to use barrier methods of contraception.

In the very long term, the development of frank or occult endometrial carcinoma arising in islands of residual endometrium remains an unresolved risk. Even women who are amenorrheic post-operatively may have foci of inactive endometrium in the uterine cavity, and there is no reason why malignant change should not take place in some cases. This risk is the reason why women with endometrial hyperplasia showing cytological or architectural atypia should not be offered endometrial resection, as they represent a high-risk group for the subsequent development of endometrial malignancy (16). Similarly, when treated patients become menopausal and develop symptoms of the climacteric-requiring estrogen replacement therapy, cyclical progestogens should be given simultaneously to protect the endometrium from overstimulation by unopposed estrogens. The theoretical risk of uterine malignancy forms an important component of our counselling process, although it may well be that the absolute risk of cancer developing in the relatively scanty remaining endometrium will prove to be less than in a control, untreated population.

CONCURRENT PROCEDURES

Hysteroscopic myomectomy is an obvious procedure to be performed during endometrial resection in women with submucous myoma, and, indeed, the resectoscope is most suited to the combined procedure. In contrast, deep intramyometrial fibroids should not be resected because of the risk of uterine perforation, excessive fluid absorption, and likely incomplete surgery. Instead, resection or rollerball ablation of the surface endometrium should suffice. It should also be remembered that hysteroscopic myomectomy on its own can be a very effective treatment for menorrhagia without the need for additional endometrial ablation (57).

Theoretically, there is no reason why TCRE should not be combined with laparoscopic pelvic surgery for endometriosis, adhesions, etc., if pelvic pain is a major component of symptomatology. However, the wisdom of such an approach instead of a definitive cure by hysterectomy with or without bilateral salpingo-oophorectomy remains to be seen. Laparoscopic sterilization, on the other hand, should be seriously considered in previously fertile women as being the most assured way to protect against an unwanted pregnancy.

CONCLUSIONS

Endometrial ablation by whatever means has offered the first real alternative to long-term drug treatment and hysterectomy for women complaining of menorrhagia (74). Of the currently available techniques, endometrial resection has a number of inherent advantages in terms of cost, speed of surgery, the ability to deal with fibroids, and the provision of tissue for histological assessment. Certainly, the early results of surgery have been encouraging, but it remains to be seen by long-term audit and randomized studies just how effective this mode of management is (75). Until then, there seems to be no reason why we should disagree with the experts and "master the challenges of the resectoscope" (76).

REFERENCES

1. Goldrath MH, Fuller TA, Segal S. Laser photovaporization of endometrium for the treatment of menorrhagia. Am J Obstet Gynecol 1981;140:14–19.

2. DeCherney A, Polan ML. Hysteroscopic management of intrauterine lesions and intractable uterine bleeding. Obstet Gynecol 1983;61: 392–397.

3. Neuwirth RS. A new technique for and additional experience with hysteroscopic resection of submucous fibroids. Am J Obstet Gynecol 1978;131:91–94.

4. Neuwirth RS. Hysteroscopic resection of submucous fibroids. Obstet Gynecol 1983:62:509–511.

5. DeCherney AH, Diamond MP, Lavy G, Polan ML. Endometrial ablation for intractable uterine bleeding: hysteroscopic resection. Obstet Gynecol 1987;70:668–669.

6. Hallez J-P, Netter A, Cariter R. Methodical intrauterine resection. Am J Obstet Gynecol 1987;156:1080–1084.

7. Magos AL, Baumann R, Turnbull AC. Transcervical resection of the endometrium in women with menorrhagia. Br Med J 1989;298:1209–1212.

8. Magos AL, Baumann R, Lockwood GM, Turnbull AC. Experience with the first 250 endometrial resections for menorrhagia. Lancet 1991;337:1074–1078.

9. Magos AL, Baumann R, Cheung K, Turnbull AC. Intrauterine surgery under intravenous sedation: an outpatient alternative to hysterectomy. Lancet 1989;ii:925–926.

10. Lockwood M, Magos AL, Baumann R, Turnbull AC. Endometrial resection when hysterectomy is undesirable, dangerous or impossible. Br J Obstet Gynaecol 1990;97:656–658.

11. Royal College of Obstetricians and Gynaecologists. Third bulletin of the audit unit. London, November 1991.

12. Chimbira TH, Anderson ABM, Turnbull AC. Relation between measured menstrual blood loss and patient's subjective assessment of loss, duration of bleeding, number of sanitary towels used, uterine weight and endometrial surface. Br J Obstet Gynaecol 1980;87:603–609.

13. Higham JM, O'Brien PMS, Shaw RW. Assessment of menstrual blood loss using a pictorial chart. Br J Obstet Gynaecol 1990;97:734–739.

14. Rees MCP. Role of menstrual blood loss measurements in management of complaints of excessive menstrual bleeding. Br J Obstet Gynaecol 1991;98:327–328.

15. Lefler HT. Premenstrual syndrome improvement after laser ablation of the endometrium for menorrhagia. J Reprod Med 1989;34:905–906.

16. Colafranceschi M, Crow J. Pathology. In: Lewis VB, Magos AL, eds. Endometrial ablation. Edinburgh: Churchill Livingstone, 1993: 183–196.

17. Rutherford AJ, Glass, MR, Wells M. Patient selection for endometrial resection. Br J Obstet Gynaecol 1991;98:228–230.

18. Fraser IS, McCarron G, Markham R, Resta T, Watts A. Measured menstrual blood loss associated with pelvic disease and coagulation disorders. Obstet Gynecol 1986;65:630–633.

19. Vancaille TG. Electrocoagulation of the endometrium with the ball-end resectoscope. Obstet Gynecol 1989;74:425–427.

20. Donnez J, Gillerot S, Bourgonjon D, Clerckx F, Nisolle M. Neodymium:YAG laser hysteroscopy in large submucous fibroids. Fertil Steril 1990;54:999–1003.

21. Loffer FD. Hysteroscopy with selective endometrial sampling compared with D&C for abnormal uterine bleeding: the value of a negative hysteroscopic view. Obstet Gynecol 1989;73:16–20.

22. Haynes PJ, Hodgson H, Anderson ABM, Turnbull AC. Measurement of menstrual blood loss in patients complaining of menorrhagia. Br J Obstet Gynaecol 1977;84:763–768.

23. Reid PC, Sharp F. Hysteroscopic Nd:YAG endometrial ablation: an in vitro and in vivo laser-tissue interaction study. Abstract from the 3rd European congress on hysteroscopy and endoscopic surgery. Amsterdam, 1988:70.

24. Loffer FD. A comparison of hysteroscopic techniques. In: Lewis VB, Magos AL, eds. Endometrial ablation. Edinburgh: Churchill Livingstone, 1993:143–150.

25. Townsend DE, Richart RM, Paskowitz RA, Woolfork RE. Rollerball coagulation the endometrium. Obstet Gynecol 1990;76:310–313.

26. Lefler HT, Sullivan GH, Hulka KJ. Modified endometrial ablation: electrocoagulation with vasopressin and suction curettage preparation. Obstet Gynecol 1991;77:949–953.

27. Garry R, Mooney P, Hasham F, Kokri M. A uterine distention system to prevent fluid absorption during Nd-YAG laser endometrial ablation. Gynaecol Endosc 1992;1:23–27.

28. Brooks PG, Serden SP, Davos I. Hormonal inhibition of the endometrium for resectoscopic endometrial ablation. Am J Obstet Gynecol 1991;161:1601–1608.

29. Magos AL, Baumann R, Turnbull AC. Safety of transcervical endometrial resection. Lancet 1990;i:44.

30. Duffy S, Reid PC, Smith JHF, Sharp F. In vitro studies of uterine electrosurgery. Obstet Gynecol 1991;78:213–220.

31. Duffy S, Reid PC, Sharp F. In vivo studies of uterine electrosurgery. Br J Obstet Gynaecol 1992;99:579–582.

32. Elliott CJR, Page VJ. Anaesthesia for endometrial ablation. In: Lewis VB, Magos AL, eds. Endometrial ablation. Edinburgh: Churchill Livingstone, 1993:57–66.

33. Lockwood GM, Baumann R, Turnbull AC, Magos AL. Extensive hysteroscopic surgery under local anaesthesia. Gynaecol Endosc 1992;1: 15–21.

34. Wood SM, Roberts FL. Air embolism during transcervical resection of endometrium. Br Med J 1990;300:945.

35. Magos AL. Endometrial resection: technique. In: Lewis VB, Magos AL, eds. Endometrial ablation. Edinburgh: Churchill Livingstone, 1993:104–115.

36. Maher PJ, Hill DJ. Transcervical endometrial resection for abnormal uterine bleeding—Report of 100 cases and review of the literature. Aust NZ J Obstet Gynaecol 1990;30;4:357–360.

37. Dwyer NA, Stirrat GM. Early endometrial carcinoma: an incidental finding after endometrial resection. Case report. Br J Obstet Gynaecol 1991;98:733–734.

38. West JH, Robinson DA. Endometrial resection and fluid absorption. Lancet 1989;ii:1387–1388.

39. Magos AL. Safety and hazards of endoscopic electrodiathermy. In: Sutton CJG, ed. New surgical techniques in gynecology. Carnforth: Parthenon Publishing, 1993:163–171.

40. Loffer FD. Endometrial ablation: where do we stand. Gynaecol Endosc 1992;1:175–179.

41. Pyper RJD, Haeri AD. A review of 80 endometrial resections for menorrhagia. Br J Obstet Gynaecol 1991;98:1049–1054.

42. Hill D, Maher P, Wood C, Lawrence A, Downing B, Lolatgis N. Complications of operative hysteroscopy. Gynaecol Endosc 1992;1: 185–189.

43. Macdonald R, Phipps J. Endometrial ablation: a safe procedure. Gynaecol Endosc 1992;1:7–9.

44. Dicker RC, Greenspan JR, Strauss LT, et al. Complications of

abdominal and vaginal hysterectomy among women of reproductive age in the United States. Am J Obstet Gynecol 1982;144: 841–848.

45. Wingo PA, Huezo CM, Rubin GL, et al. The mortality risk associated with hysterectomy. Am J Obstet Gynecol 1985;152:803–808.

46. Centerwall BS. Premenopausal hysterectomy and cardiovascular disease. Am J Obstet Gynecol 1981;139:58–61.

47. Siddle N, Sarrel P, Whitehead MI. The effect of hysterectomy on the age of ovarian failure: identification of a subgroup of women with premature loss of ovarian function and literature review. Fertil Steril 1987;47:94–100.

48. Taylor T, Smith AN, Fulton PM. Effect of hysterectomy on bowel function. Br Med J 1989;299:300–301.

49. Broadbent JAM, Molnar BG, Cooper MJW, Magos AL. Endoscopic management of uterine perforation occurring during endometrial resection. Br J Obstet Gynaecol 1992;99:1018.

50. Vulgaropulos SP, Haley LC, Hulka JF. Intrauterine pressure and fluid absorption during continuous flow hysterectomy. Am J Obstet Gynecol 1992;167:386–391.

51. Molnar BG, Broadbent JAM, Magos AL. Fluid overload risk score for endometrial resection. Gynaecol Endosc 1992;1:133–138.

52. Baumann R, Magos AL, Kay JDS, Turnbull AC. Absorption of glycine irrigating solution during transcervical resection of the endometrium. Br Med J 1990;300:304–305.

53. Boubli L, Blanc M, Bautrand E, et al. Le risque metabolique de la chirurgie hysteroscopique. J Gynecol Obstet Biol Reprod 1990;19: 217–222.

54. Byers GF, Pinion S, Parkin DE, Chambers WA. Fluid absorption during transcervical resection of the endometrium. Gynaecol Endosc 1993;2:21–23.

55. Istre O, Skajaa K, Schjoensby AP, Forman A. Change in serum electrolytes after transcervical resection of endometrium and submucous fibroids with use of glycine for uterine irrigation. Obstet Gynecol 1992;80:218–222.

56. Duffy S, Cruise M, Reilly C, Reid PC, Sharp F. Ethanol labeling: detection of early fluid absorption in endometrial resection. Obstet Gynecol 1992;79:300–304.

57. Derman SG, Rehnstrom J, Neuwirth RS. The long-term effectiveness

of hysteroscopic treatment of menorrhagia and leiomyomas. Obstet Gynecol 1991;77:591–594.

58. Van Damme JP. One stage endometrial ablation: results in 200 cases. Eur J Obstet Gynaecol Reprod Biol 1992;434:209–214.

59. Broadbent JAM, Magos AL. Endometrial resection: results and complications. In: Lewis VB, Magos AL, eds. Endometrial ablation. Edinburgh: Churchill Livingstone, 1993:115–131.

59. Hill DJ, Maher PJ. Intrauterine surgery using electrocautery. Aust NZ J Obstet Gynaecol 1990;30:145–146.

60. Rankin L, Steinberg LH. Transcervical resection of the endometrium: a review of 400 consecutive patients. Br J Obstet Gynaecol 1992;99: 911–914.

61. Browning JJ, Pardey JM, Anderson RS, Barley VL. Endometrial resection after radiotherapy for cervical carcinoma. Int J Gynecol Obstet 1991;36:243–245.

62. Cooper MJW, Magos AL, Baumann R, Rees MCP. The effect of endometrial resection of menstrual blood loss. Gynaecol Endosc 1992;1:195–198.

63. McLure N, Mamers PM, Healy DL, Hill DJ, Lawrence AS, Wingfield M, Paterson PJ. A quantitative assessment of endometrial electrocautery in the management of menorrhagia and a comparative report of argon laser endometrial ablation. Gynaecol Endosc 1992;1:199–202.

64. Still RM, Walsh DJ. A pilot study to assess the learning curve in transcervical endometrial resection; possible implications for postgraduate accreditation. Gynaecol Endosc 1992;1:111–113.

65. Gannon MJ, Holt EM, Fairbank J, Fitzgerald M, Milne MA, Crystal AM, Greenhalf JO. A randomised trial comparing endometrial resection and abdominal hysterectomy for the treatment of menorrhagia. Br Med J 1991;303:1362–1364.

66. Dwyer N, Hutton J, Stirrat GM. Randomised controlled trial comparing endometrial resection with abdominal hysterectomy for the surgical treatment of menorrhagia. Br J Obstet Gynaecol 1993;100: 237–243.

67. Sculpher MJ, Bryan S, Dwyer N, Hutton J, Stirrat GM. An economic evaluation of transcervical endometrial resection versus abdominal hysterectomy for the treatment of menorrhagia. Br J Obstet Gynaecol 1993;100:244–252.

68. Hill DJ, Maher PJ, Wood CW, Davison G. Haematometra—a compli-

cation of endometrial resection. Aust NZ J Obstet Gynaecol 1992;32: 285–286.

69. Ashworth MT, Moss CI, Kenyon WE. Granulomatous endometritis following hysteroscopic resection of the endometrium. Histopath 1991;18:185–187.

70. Ferryman SR, Stephens, Gough D. Necrotising granulomatous endometritis following endometrial ablation therapy. Br J Obstet Gynaecol 1992;99:928–930.

71. Hill DJ, Maher PJ. Pregnancy following endometrial ablation. Gynaecol Endosc 1992;1:47–49.

72. Whitelaw NL, Garry R, Sutton CJG. Pregnancy following endometrial ablation: 2 case reports. Gynaecol Endosc 1992;1:129–132.

73. Lam AM, Al-Jumaily RY, Holt EM. Ruptured ectopic pregnancy in an amenorrhoeic woman after transcervical resection of the endometrium. Aust NZ J Obstet Gynaecol 1992;32:81–82.

74. Magos AL. Management of menorrhagia. Br Med J 1990;300:1537–1538.

75. Coulter A. Managing menorrhagia with endometrial resection. Lancet 1993;341:1185–1186.

76. Brooks PG, DeCherney AH, Loffer FD, Neuwirth RS. Resectoscopy: mastering the challenges. Contemp Ob Gyn 1989;34:131–148.

13

Role of Second-look Resectoscope and Repeat Procedures

Richard J. Gimpelson

Second-look or repeat resectoscope procedures are indicated under three circumstances: 1) when initial endometrial ablation fails to control menorrhagia (1), 2) when a submucous or intramural leiomyoma is only partially resected (2,3) and is symptomatic, or 3) when a new fibroid develops (2,3).

ENDOMETRIAL ABLATION

Anatomy

When attempting a repeat endometrial ablation, one must be aware of the uterine anatomy. The cavity is usually a different shape than an unablated cavity. The shape is narrow and cylindrical, cornua are usually obliterated, and myometrium may be thinner. The uterus usually sounds to a shorter depth following endometrial ablation. Occasionally, the cavity is interlaced with synechiae (Figures 13-1, 13-2).

Indications

Repeat endometrial ablation is indicated whenever there is a failure to achieve the desired results from an initial endometrial ablation. Patients undergoing repeat ablation fall into one of five categories (1):

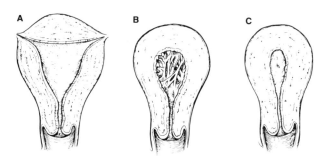

FIGURE 13-1

Drawings of uterus: (A) normal uterine cavity; (B) postablation (synechiae); (C) postablation (narrowed and cylindrical).

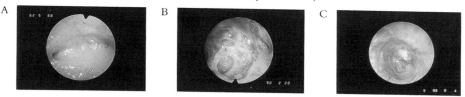

FIGURE 13-2

Photos of uterus: (A) normal cavity; (B) postablation (synechiae); (C) postablation (narrowed and cylindrical).

1. Improved but still heavy or prolonged flow,
2. Initial procedure not completed because of leiomyomas,
3. Physical or mental disability with amenorrhea desired,
4. Amenorrhea desired by patient despite achieving normal or light flow,
5. Unimproved.

Most patients will fall into the "improved but still heavy or prolonged flow" category. It is recommended that a 6-month interval be observed before repeat ablation is performed to allow for full healing of the uterus and also to allow for a recognizable and definable menstrual pattern.

Methods

Both roller electrode and Nd–YAG laser have been used for repeat ablation (1). Repeat ablation with the laser affords the advantage of fitting the laser fiber through a conventional 21 French operating hysteroscope and more easily entering the constricted uterine cavity. However, with increasing use of electrosurgical techniques, increasing experience with resectoscopic repeat ablations is obtained.

Surgical Technique

After allowing for the 6-month recovery period following initial endometrial ablation (4), a patient can be scheduled for repeat endometrial ablation. If it has been over one year since the initial ablation, the endometrium must be re-evaluated to rule out cancer or precancerous changes. Suppression of the endometrium is achieved either by medical suppression [Danocrine 800 mg/day for 4 weeks (5), or GnRH agonist for 6 weeks (6)] or by mechanical preparation [suction curettage with a 7-mm suction curette (7,8)] (Figure 13-3). Mechanical preparation is carried out for 2 to 2½ minutes just prior to the ablation.

The mechanical preparation of the endometrium makes repeat ablation more convenient and comfortable for the patient since sur-

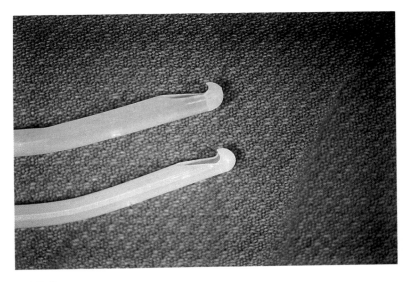

FIGURE 13-3

7 French suction curette.

gery can be scheduled without specific time requirements or delays and the patient is free from side effects of endometrial suppression medications. Uterine entry is easier when a nonatrophic state is present, as is the case with mechanical preparation.

The patient is given general anesthesia, epidural anesthesia, or local anesthesia with sedation. A paracervical block with 0.25% bupivacaine may make cervical dilatation easier and less uncomfortable. Pitressin (2 units/10cc) may be concurrently administered to reduce fluid absorption and bleeding, but is not without risk (see Chapter 14). This paracervical block is given even with general and regional anesthesia to reduce postoperative discomfort.

Just as with other procedures using high-flow, low viscosity liquids, the fluid inflow and outflow must be monitored very closely. Initial entry into the uterus is with a 5-mm diagnostic sheath and 4-mm telescope. Entry is usually achieved without the need for dilators. Following this initial entry, a continuous flow operating hysteroscope (21 French) can be inserted 90% of the time, again without need for dilators. Use of the diagnostic sheath reduces the number of blind insertions into the uterus and reduces the risk of perforation. At this point, the suction curettage is performed if medical preparation of the endometrium has not been utilized (Figures 13-3, 13-4). If the resectoscope is to be used, further cervical dilatation is usually performed at this time.

Usually, lactated Ringer's is used with the Nd-YAG laser. However, electrolyte-free fluids must be used with the resectoscope (see

A 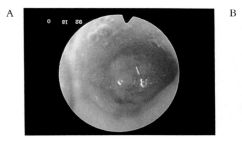 B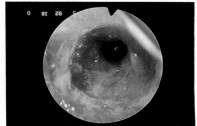

FIGURE 13-4

Uterine cavity before (A) and after (B) curettage.

Role of Second-look Resectoscope and Repeat Procedures 257

Chapter 5). The power is set at 50 to 55 W for the Nd–YAG laser, and a nontouch technique allows the procedure to be performed in 10 to 15 minutes. Approximately the same amount of time is used with the roller electrode set at 60 W coagulating current or 80 W cutting circuit. With either modality, the technique involves ablation from the fundus toward the internal os to enhance the success of the procedure and reduce the risk of perforation. Once the procedure is completed, the patient is observed and almost always discharged on the same day of surgery.

Although most ablations are now being performed with the roller electrode or loop electrode rather than the Nd–YAG laser, it is the opinion of the author that repeat ablation is more easily accomplished with the Nd–YAG laser. The reason is that a laser fiber will go through a 21 French hysteroscope sheath, whereas the roller or loop electrode requires a minimum 24 French sheath. Since the uterine cavity is usually shortened and narrowed with a cylindrical shape following endometrial ablation, a 21 French sheath is easier to insert than a 24 French sheath. However, if one prefers the roller electrode for repeat ablation, it is most likely the results will be comparable to those from the laser.

Risks

The risks of repeat endometrial ablation are the same as those for initial endometrial ablation (9): fluid overload, perforation, bleeding, infection, and thermal injury to structures outside the uterus.

Fluid overload is avoided by carefully monitoring fluid inflow and outflow throughout the procedure. A sheet for keeping track has been utilized for ease of record keeping (Figure 13-5). Electrolytes are obtained prior to the procedure and absorption of fluid is limited to 1500 cc lactated Ringer's or 1000 cc electrolyte-free solution. However, more rigid limits are used depending on the medical condition of the patient. Usually, observation or Lasix is used for excess fluids. If larger levels of fluids are somehow absorbed, full intensive care therapy may be needed.

Perforation is more likely to occur with blind insertion of dilators and sounds rather than the hysteroscope or resectoscope. Such a risk

HYSTEROSCOPIC SURGERY
FLUIDS
INTAKE AND OUTPUT

FLOW SHEET

TIME (q 10 Min)	FLUID IN	FLUID OUT	PUMP PRESSURE	COMMENTS
TOTAL				
OTHER FLUIDS				
I.V.s:				
Urine:				

FIGURE 13-5

Sheet for monitoring fluid use.

may be higher in patients undergoing a secondary procedure. Theoretically, the smaller cavity may predispose patients to a perforation. If perforation occurs, with the diagnostic sheath, dilator, or sound, the procedure is ended and observation is all that is needed. A repeat procedure can be performed in approximately 3 months, after healing has occurred. If perforation occurs with the operating hysteroscope or resectoscope, laparoscopy may be utilized to assess the damage. If the laser or electrical generator was being operated when perforation occured, then laparotomy would usually need to be performed to evaluate damage to bowel, bladder, or vessels.

The most serious type of injury would be an unrecognized

thermal injury to abdominal structures without perforation of the uterus. This occurence can be minimized by avoiding powers above 55 W with the Nd-YAG laser and continually moving the tip across the uterus to avoid constant exposure in one area. The roller electrode should also be kept moving to avoid similar problems. Powers for the electrical method have not been as well studied as laser, but 60 W coagulating and 80 W cutting current have accomplished satisfactory results in the author's practice.

Postoperative Management

Postoperative discomfort is usually easily controlled with mild analgesia, such as nonsteroidal anti-inflammatory agents. Patients are given a home instruction sheet (Figure 13-6) and instructed to return in one month for uterine sounding and cervical dilatation to reduce the potential for developing hematometra secondary to cervical stenosis.

Results

Early studies of endometrial ablation with the Nd-YAG laser demonstrated that repeat ablation would be successful most of the time

Postoperative Instructions
for
Endometrial Ablation

- You should rest this evening.
- Avoid alcoholic beverages for about 48 hours.
- Avoid intercourse for about 72 hours.
- You will need to make an appointment to be seen in my office one month from the surgery for a follow-up examination, uterine sounding, and hemoglobin/hematocrit.
- You should notify me if any of the following occurs:
  - Fever above 101 degrees
  - Severe pains
  - Bleeding that requires more pads than a usual period. You will expect some drainage and some bleeding that may continue for 4 to 6 weeks
- You may experience moderate to severe cramping lasting 48–72 hours that should respond to pain medication prescribed.

FIGURE 13-6

Postablation instruction sheet.

ablation is a viable option with expected good or excellent results most of the time.

Whether the Nd–YAG laser, roller electrode, or loop electrode is utilized for endometrial ablation (Table 13-1), a small number of patients will not achieve satisfactory results with the initial procedure. However, with repeat ablation, most patients will be satisfied with the outcome and not need further treatment (11).

Since the author's paper was published (1), an additional 69 patients have undergone initial endometrial ablation. Only two additional repeat ablations have been performed in the same time period for a total of 18 repeat ablations out of 212 patients. Amenorrhea was achieved in 12 of the 18 repeat ablations.

Only one patient who underwent repeat ablation had a subsequent hysterectomy and was found to have a leiomyoma and simple

TABLE 13-1

Author	Number of Patients	Repeat Procedures (Success/Total)	Initial Technique	Repeat Technique
Goldrath (10)	216	3/4	Nd-YAG	Nd-YAG
Loffer (11)	36	2/2	Nd-YAG	Nd-YAG
Garry et al. (13)	479	26/39	Nd-YAG	Nd-YAG
			or	or
Magos et al. (14)	234	13/16	Roller	Roller
			Loop	Loop
Leffler, et al. (7)	38	2/2	Nd-YAG	Roller
			or	
			Roller	
Gimpelson et al. (1)	143	16/16	Nd-YAG	Nd-YAG
			or	or
			Roller	Roller
Rankin et al. (15)	400	28/31*	Loop or	Loop or
			Roller	Roller
Total	1,546	90/110		

*One patient had three procedures before success

hyperplasia. An additional five of the 212 patients had a change in their menstrual pattern that occurred over one year following endometrial ablation and were evaluated by hysteroscopy and curettage. All findings were benign, and since flow was well within an acceptable range, no repeat ablation was performed. The uterine cavities in these patients had the same scarred and constricted appearance as the patients undergoing repeat ablation.

Three patients who have gone through menopause (documented by elevated follicle-stimulating hormone [FSH] and decreased estradiol) have been hysteroscoped prior to estrogen replacement therapy and also had the typical postablation appearance of the uterine cavity.

LEIOMYOMAS

Indications

Leiomyomas with large intramural components can often be removed by multistage operations at intervals of one month or more if they cannot be completely removed at the initial procedure. Infertility or continous bleeding are two indications that leiomyomas remain (2,3,16), warranting second-look resectoscopic surgery. When fertility is of concern, a final procedure is performed to eliminate any synechiae that may have developed from use of the resectoscope.

Methods

Scissors, Nd–YAG laser, and resectoscope can all be utilized; however, the resectoscope is the quickest modality. An instrument of extreme value for myomectomy is the Corson Myoma Grasping Forceps (Figure 13-7). Its strong jaws can tightly grip a leiomyoma gently and completely extract it out of the myometrial bed and out through the cervical canal.

Surgical Procedure

When a leiomyoma with a large intramural component has been partially resected until flush with the endometrium, the next step

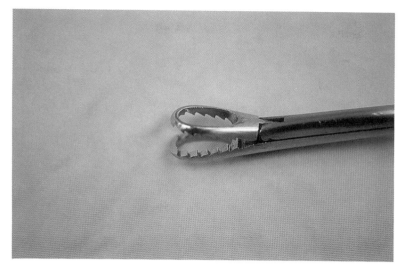

FIGURE 13-7

Corson Myoma Grasping Forceps.

to remove the instruments from the uterine cavity and wait several minutes. On re-examination, the leiomyoma will often rise out of the myometrium and be in a position for further resection or extraction. If the myoma does not rise out of the myometrium, one can terminate the procedure and re-evaluate the cavity via hysterosalpingogram or office hysteroscopy several months after the procedure. If a residual myoma is seen, the patient may be brought to the operating room at that time. At this follow-up procedure, the leiomyoma has usually delivered a large portion of itself into the uterine cavity and can be once more partially or totally resected. If only partial resection is achieved, the scenario is repeated and the patient can be brought back again. This method has allowed the removal of quite large leiomyomas with ease (Figure 13-8).

Risks

The risks for resection of leiomyomas are the same as those of any hysteroscopic procedure as described earlier in this chapter. In addi-

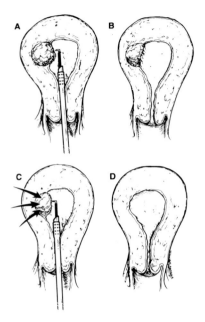

FIGURE 13-8

Drawing of myoma migration. (A) Submucous leiomyoma with significant intramural component; (B) resection of leiomyoma to level of endometrium; (C) migration of leiomyoma toward uterine cavity; (D) complete resection of leiomyoma.

tion, there are certain risks that are increased with myomectomy. Gonadotropin-releasing hormone agonists can often be utilized to shrink leiomyomas, stop bleeding, and allow for the migration of the intramural segment of the myoma into the uterine cavity as the myometrium shrinks and compresses the myoma (17). However, the GnRH agonists have risks that must be addressed (18). Since the uterus will shrink more than the myoma, a tumor filling half the uterine cavity prior to GnRH agonists may well fill the entire uterine cavity after a course of GnRH agonists and actually make resection of the myoma more difficult. Also, heavy uterine bleeding has been reported on occasion when GnRH agonists are used with leiomyomas (3).

Uterine perforation may occur with too vigorous a resection or attempts at extraction before the myometrium can push the leiomyoma into the uterine cavity. If visualization becomes uncorrectably poor and intrauterine pressure diminishes, one may suspect perforation, and laparotomy or laparoscopy should be considered to assess and correct the problem. Transvaginal ultrasound prior to myomectomy and repeat procedures will give an estimate of myometrical thickness overlying the leiomyoma (19). Occasionally, bleeding is encountered, but is often limited as the uterus spontaneously contracts. If bleeding is persistent, a catheter can be inserted into the uterus and the balloon distended for several hours as a tamponade.

Fluid overload is more a concern with myomectomy than with endometrial ablation because the electrical loop used for myomectomy is more likely to expose the uterine vasculature than ablation with roller electrode (3). Safety measures include preoperative electrolytes, close monitoring of fluids, and termination of the procedure if a 1000-cc deficit occurs. The same sheet used for monitoring fluids with endometrial ablation is used for monitoring fluids for myomectomy and all other hysteroscopic procedures in which low viscosity liquids are used.

Postoperative Management

Postoperative patients are usually discharged on the day of surgery and instructed to return in one week for a follow-up visit. They are given a going home instruction sheet for guidance (Figure 13-9). Antibiotics are sometimes used, and after complete myomectomy, a 3-week course of estrogen is used to stimulate endometrial growth when infertility is a concern.

The resectoscope is far superior to laser or scissors in ease of use, speed of surgery, and thoroughness of removal. The author has abandoned use of the Nd-YAG laser for myomectomy, especially in combination with endometrial ablation because of the lengthy operating times and large amount of fluid absorbed (12). Scissors are fine for small leiomyomas and for office use but are too slow compared to the resectoscope and loop electrode in the operating room.

Postoperative Instructions
for
Hysteroscopic Myomectomy

- You should rest this evening.
- Avoid alcoholic beverages for about 48 hours.
- Avoid intercourse for about 72 hours.
- You will need to make an appointment to be seen in my office in one week for follow-up examination.
- You should notify me if any of the following occurs:
  - Fever above 101 degrees
  - Severe pains
  - Bleeding that requires more pads than a usual period.
- You may experience moderate to severe cramping lasting 48–72 hours that should respond to over the counter ibuprofen or pain medication that may have been prescribed.

FIGURE 13-9

Postmyomectomy instruction sheet.

CLINICAL PEARLS

✖ One should not hesitate to offer repeat endometrial ablation because the outcome is usually excellent.

✖ If there is a change in postablation menstrual pattern, this should be evaluated just like initial abnormal bleeding.

✖ The previous ablated cavity is smaller than the original uterine cavity.

✖ The Nd-YAG laser may be easier to use during repeat procedures as it only requires a 21 French instrument.

✖ Do transvaginal ultrasound prior to myomectomy to assess the myometrium overlying the leiomyoma.

✖ If a leiomyoma is partially resected, remove all instruments, wait several minutes, and reinsert the resectoscope to see if the leiomyoma has risen out of the myometrium. If it has, finish the procedure. If it has not, discharge the patient and re-evaluate in one month. The leiomyoma will almost always be visible and resectable.

REFERENCES

1. Gimpelson RJ, Kaigh J. Endometrial ablation repeat procedures. J Reprod Med 1992;37:629–635

2. Brooks PG, Loffer FD, Serden SP. Resectoscopic removal of symptomatic intrauterine lesions. J Reprod Med 1989;34:435–437.

3. Indman PD. Hysteroscopic treatment of menorrhagia associated with uterine leiomyomas. Obstet Gynecol 1993;81:716–720.

4. Goldrath MH, Fuller TA, Segal S. Laser photovaporization of the endometrium for the treatment of menorrhagia. Am J Obstet Gynecol 1981;140:14–19.

5. Goldrath MH. Use of danazol in hysteroscopic surgery for menorrhagia. J Reprod Med 1990;35:91–96.

6. Brooks PG, Serden SP, Davos I. Hormonal inhibition of the endometrium for resectoscopic endometrial ablation. Am J Obstet Gynecol 1991;164:1601–1608.

7. Lefler HT, Sullivan GH, Hulka JF. Modified endometrial ablation: electrocoagulation with vasopressin and suction curettage preparation. Obstet Gynecol 1991;77:949–953.

8. Gimpelson RJ, Kaigh J. Mechanical preparation of the endometrium prior to endometrial ablation. J Reprod Med 1992;37:691–694.

9. Brooks PG. Complications of operative hysteroscopy: how safe is it? Clin Obstet Gynecol 1992;35:256–261.

10. Goldrath MH. Hysteroscopic laser surgery. In: Baggish MS, ed. Basic and advanced laser surgery in gynecology. Norwalk, CT: Appleton-Century-Crofts, 1985: 357–372.

11. Loffer FD. Hysteroscopic endometrial ablation with the Nd:YAG laser using a nontouch technique. Obstet Gynecol 1987;69:679–682.

12. Gimpelson RJ. Hysteroscopic Nd:YAG laser ablation of the endometrium. J Reprod Med 1988;33:872–876.

13. Garry R, Erian J, Grochmal SA. A multi-centre collaborative study into the treatment of menorrhagia by Nd:YAG laser ablation of the endometrium. Br J Obstet Gynaecol 1991;98:357–362.

14. Magos AL, Baumann R, Lockwood GM, Turnbull AC. Experience with the first 250 endometrial resections for menorrhagia. Lancet 1991;337:1074–1078.

15. Rankin L, Steinberg LH. Transcervical resection of the endometrium:

a review of 400 consecutive cases. Br J Obstet Gynaecol 1992;99:911–914.

16. Derman SG, Rehnstrom J, Neuwirth RS. The long-term effectiveness of hysteroscopic treatment of menorrhagia and leiomyomas. Obstet Gynecol 1991;77:591–594.

17. Friedman AJ, Barbieri RL. Leuprolide acetate: applications in gynecology. Curr Probl Obstet Gynecol Fertil 1988;11:205–236.

18. Friedman AJ, Juneau-Norcross M, Rein MS. Adverse effects of leuprolide acetate depot treatment. Fertil Steril 1993;59:448–450.

19. Batzer FR. Vaginosonographic evaluation of the nonpregnant uterus. Am J Gynecol Health 1992;6:28–31.

14

Complications of Operative Hysteroscopy

Philip G. Brooks

O perative hysteroscopy generally comprises procedures that are relatively simple and safe, resulting in few complications. In a recent survey of its members conducted by the American Association of Gynecologic Laparoscopists, the overall complication rate for almost 14,000 hysteroscopic procedures performed by the respondents in 1988 was reported as 2%, with major complications (perforation, hemorrhage, fluid overload, bowel or urinary tract injury) occurring in less than 1% of procedures (1).

This chapter describes the complications seen during or subsequent to operative hysteroscopy. They include trauma, hemorrhage, distention media–related, infections, risk of subsequent pregnancy, thermal injury, cervical stenosis and hematometria, and the conceptual risk of endometrial cancer. It will also attempt to elucidate the reasons for the complications and outline steps to avoid them, if possible, and to manage them when they occur.

TRAUMATIC COMPLICATIONS

Inserting rigid instruments through the soft cervical canal and into a hollow organ like the uterus are maneuvers that will occasionally result in traumatic lacerations or bleeding. This is especially a problem if the cervix has to be dilated enough to pass wider caliber operating instruments. Careful placement of tenacula and gentle dilatation of the cervix minimize these risks. The use of laminaria tents is favored by some hysteroscopists but is avoided by others because of the possibility that overdilation will occur, resulting in loss of distention medium and intrauterine pressure, in turn producing poor visualization. In addition, anecdotal cases of endometritis or purulent cervicitis have been reported subsequent to the use of laminaria, but this has not been supported scientifically.

While too low an intrauterine pressure can result in poor visualization, excessive pressures are also harmful. They will increase the risk of fluid overload due to intravascular intravasation; this is especially a problem if salt-poor distention media are used. It will also increase the risk of gas embolization, when a gaseous distention medium is used. Fortunately, this is very unlikely at flow rates routinely used for CO_2 hysteroscopy. Great care must be taken if instillation of distending media (such as high molecular weight dextran) is performed manually with syringes. The proper technique should be to infuse the medium slowly and hold the pressure steady without injecting more fluid, as long as visualization is adequate. This is where working off a video monitor with a video camera attached to the hysteroscope is especially advantageous as both the operator and the assistant infusing the medium can see the view and the procedure simultaneously.

Rupture of the oviducts from excessive gas pressures with or without bilateral hydrosalpinx has been reported anecdotally. This usually results from use of the wrong equipment or excessive insufflation pressures. It is imperative that only insufflators designed exclusively for hysteroscopy be used for uterine distention. Hysteroscopic insufflators are designed to produce flow rates of only 100 to 200 mL per minute (although flow rates of 40 to 60 mL per minute are almost always sufficient). Most laparoscopic insufflators, even older models, deliver between 1000 and 3000 mL per minute. A case was reported where, due to a lack of available equipment, a carbon dioxide tank was attached directly to a hysteroscope without any insufflator with governors, etc. This resulted not only in the rupture of normal oviducts but also the rupture of the patient's diaphragm, resulting in massive pneumothorax, cardiac arrest, and death (2).

In addition to restricting flow rates, the hysteroscopist should also use equipment that can be set to deliver pressures under 100 mmHg. The basic physiology is that, once the intrauterine surgery opens sinuses and venous channels, gas or fluid will flow into the vascular tree when the intrauterine pressure exceeds the intravascular pressure in the vessel open to the endometrial cavity.

Perforation of the uterus is a well documented risk of operative hysteroscopy, with most hysteroscopists encountering it at one time or another. Lomano reported one perforation of the uterus in 61 laser endometrial ablation procedures, while Goldrath reported it once in his first 196 laser ablations (3,4). We reported one perforation in 216 uterine resectoscopic operations involving both resections of intrauterine growths and ablations (5), and, at the time of this writing, still have had only one in almost 500 resectoscopic procedures.

Most perforations result in little or no serious bleeding or other problems but often require a diagnostic laparoscopy to ensure that there is no damage to adherent or adjacent structures and that there is no unsuspected laceration of large blood vessels. As such, when operative hysteroscopy is scheduled, all patients should have given prior consent for laparoscopy. More about the use of concomitant laparoscopy to avoid or manage complications of hysteroscopy will be discussed at the end of this chapter.

HEMORRHAGIC COMPLICATIONS

Intraoperative bleeding other than from lacerations due to forceful dilation or tenaculum tears, as noted above, occurs infrequently and usually is the result of inadvertent or unintentional trauma to the uterine wall. It can occur from lacerations or false passages created during either the dilation of the cervix or the insertion of the hysteroscope and sheath through the endocervical canal.

In addition, excessive bleeding can occur after operative procedures, such as the incision of uterine septae or synechiae, especially when deep penetration into healthy myometrium occurs. This can be done whether using mechanical methods (scissors) or with electrical or laser energy, although using either of the latter two is usually associated with coagulation of the smaller vessels.

Intraoperative bleeding sufficent to require intrauterine tamponade with a Foley catheter or a balloon catheter specially designed for intrauterine use by Neuwirth, was reported in nine out of 40 (22.5%) resectoscopic procedures by DeCherney and colleagues (6), one out of every three resectoscopic cases by Neuwirth (personal communication), and four of the first 216 cases in our series (1.9%) (5–7).

The technique we use for intrauterine tamponade is the placement of the balloon into the uterine cavity in the operating room (often performing a paracervical block with a longer acting anesthetic drug to minimize the cramping postoperatively) and filling the balloon with approximately 10 to 15 mL of liquid (saline, water, etc.) until moderate resistance is felt. After about an hour, half of the liquid is removed. If no bleeding occurs over the next hour, the rest of the liquid is removed, but the catheter is left in the uterine cavity. If no bleeding is encountered over the next hour, the catheter is removed and the patient is usually discharged. If active bleeding recurs at any time prior to removal of the catheter, it is reinflated and left in place for a longer period, often overnight.

To minimize bleeding during postoperative procedures, it is our practice to inject about four to six units of Pitressin, diluted ten units per 20 mL of saline, directly into the cervical stroma prior to each procedure. Care must be taken to avoid intravascular injection, which can cause significant cardiovascular changes. The small amount of Pitressin decreases the likelihood of systemic reactions. In a recent double-blind, randomized, prospective study, Corson and colleagues showed a statistically significant reduction in blood loss and amount of intravasation of distending media (sorbitol or glycine) when Pitressin was used as contrasted with placebo (7).

Townsend has reported on the use of a vasopressin-soaked pack in 17 women with refractory bleeding after submucous myoma resection (8). A 1-inch gauge pack was soaked in a solution of 20 units

Pitressin and 30 cc saline solution. The pack was then placed in the uterine cavity by forceps and left for no more than one hour. Resolution of bleeding without significant systemic side effects was noted in all patients.

Preoperative medical therapy has been used to decrease the thickness and vascularity of the endometrium or to shrink myomata. Such therapy reduces the risk of bleeding and makes the procedure easier to perform (see Chapter 7). Of all the drugs used for this purpose, we prefer using a GnRH analog, leuprolide acetate depot, for a minimum of 4 weeks prior to the procedure (9,10), although Danocrine and progestins have been used by others (1). Our experience with the latter two drugs is that the endometrium is often fluffier, more deciduous, and more vascular as confirmed histologically. On microscopic examination, after the use of GnRH analogs for at least 3 to 4 weeks, the endometrium is thinner, more compact, markedly devoid of intra- and extracellular fluid, and contains fewer and more inactive glands and smaller and fewer blood vessels.

DISTENTION MEDIUM HAZARDS

Complications specifically related to distention media were reported to have occurred in less than 4% of cases in a retrospective survey (1).

Carbon Dioxide

Embolism is the most feared complication from the use of CO_2 as a distention medium. Fortunately, when the principles of low flow and low pressure, i.e., using a hysteroflator only, are followed, the risks are very low.

Two studies, one with dogs (12) and one with sheep (3), both showed that, even with infusion of the gas directly into the femoral veins of these animals, CO_2 produces very few systemic cardiovascular problems unless the flow rates were higher than those recommended for hysteroscopy and for longer periods of time. Thus, when CO_2 is the distending medium chosen, the margin of safety is quite wide. Several reports of fatal CO_2 embolization during operative hysteroscopy (14,15) have appeared in the literature. These resulted from the inappropriate use of CO_2-cooled laser fibers with sapphire tips for intrauterine operative procedures. The problem occurred because the flow rates of CO_2 for cooling laser tips are equivalent to that of a laparoflator, or greater than one liter per minute, thus over ten times greater than the flow rates recommended for hysteroscopy. As a result of these reports, the FDA has issued a warning never to use gas-cooled laser fibers or tips for intrauterine surgery (16).

High Molecular Weight dextran (Hyskon)

A major complication from the use of dextran 70, although very rare, is that of anaphylactic shock. No data exist regarding the frequency of this problem, and reports are sporadic and anecdotal. It is believed to be an immunologic reaction and can be prevented, according to Renck (17), by the intravenous injection of a small amount of 15% dextran two minutes prior to the use of dextran 70. However, very few hysteroscopists using dextran 70 consider the risk serious enough to warrant this method of prophylaxis routinely.

Although still uncommon, a more frequent problem resulting from the use of dextran 70 as distention medium may occur when a substantial volume is retained in the patient, due to intravascular intravasation via open vessels or sinuses.

The potential for dextran 70 osmotically to draw in large volumes of water may result in ascites when the fluid is in the peritoneal cavity or fluid overload when excessive Hyskon enters the vascular tree. When this occurs, careful use of diuretics and electrolyte management may be required. Coagulation abnormalities may also be associated with Hyskon use (see Chapter 5). Prevention is most important and is accomplished by limiting the amount of dextran used during a procedure and carefully monitoring the volume retained in the patient, i.e., assessing the amount used less the amount retrieved at the end of the procedure. One note of medicolegal importance: the package insert provided by the manufacturer of dextran 70 states that no more than 500 mL of this liquid should ever be used during operative hysteroscopy. It would be difficult to defend if more liquid was used and the patient developed a serious problem, even if it can be shown that much of the liquid ran out onto the floor or drapes.

Low Viscosity Liquid Complications

Low viscosity fluids, such as sorbitol, glycine, mannitol, dextrose in water, etc., which are used primarily with intrauterine electrosurgical (resectoscopic) procedures, may result in significant hyponatremia and fluid overload when retained in the patient because they are sodium-free. In our experience, retention of these fluids mainly occurs from intravasation resulting from opening into large venous sinuses during the operative procedure or from lacerations or false passages produced during a difficult dilatation of the cervix. It is mandatory to monitor intake and output of these liquids during and after each procedure, with the immediate assessment of serum electrolytes if a discrepancy of 1000 mL or more occurs in the healthy patient or 750 mL in the older patient and/or in those with a history of cardiovascular compromise (a flow sheet for fluid monitoring is found in Chapter 13).

If hyponatremia (serum sodium <125 mg) or fluid overload occurs, it is strongly recommended that the surgeon *stop the procedure* immediately and consider completing it in the near future. The use of diuretics and restriction of intravenous fluids may be necessary. To re-emphasize prevention of this very serious problem, it is essential to monitor the inflow and outflow volumes of these liquids when they are used for distention during operative hysteroscopy.

In addition to the hyponatremia that results from excessive intravasation of low viscosity liquids, there are scattered reports of central nervous system toxicity from glycine, mainly in the urologic (18) and orthopedic (19) literature. A syndrome including encephalopathy and transient blindness has been reported after transurethral prostatectomy and after electrosurgical arthroscopic procedures associated with the use of glycine as an irrigation medium and wherein very high levels of serum glycine and its metabolic byproduct, ammonia, are detected. No such syndrome has been reported after the use of glycine for gynecologic resectoscopic procedures, but again, careful monitoring of inflow and outflow volumes is essential to prevent the retention of too much distention medium fluid in the patient's vascular tree.

INFECTION

Endometritis is an occasional complication following hysteroscopy, occurring in one out of 4000 cases performed by Salat-Baroux (20) and in two of 216 patients in our series (5). When it occurs, it is usually following longer operative procedures, especially with repeated insertion and removal of the hysteroscope through the cervical canal. Endometritis, in our experience, is usually treated with oral antibiotics and rarely requires hospitalization. To prevent it from occurring, the use of prophylactic antibiotics is recommended when long procedures are contemplated, as well as for all patients being treated for infertility.

McCausland and coworkers (21) reported that out of 200 cases of operative hysteroscopy where no prophylactic antibiotics were used, three of the patients with a history of pelvic inflammatory disease (PID) developed tubo-ovarian abscesses, whereas no cases were seen in 500 patients treated prophylactically prior to and immediately after the procedure. In addition, it may be appropriate to obtain cervical cultures prior to hysteroscopy when the patient's past history (or additional high-risk factors) suggests a possible risk for infection.

Finally, while extremely uncommon, a flareup of PID has been reported (even after diagnostic hysteroscopy), occurring in one of a series of 34 such diagnostic procedures reported by Cohen (22).

PREGNANCY FOLLOWING ABLATION

Pregnancies have been reported following endometrial ablation by laser, resection, and coagulation (23,24). Because of known obstetric complications in patients with Asherman's syndrome, there has been appropriate concern regarding obstetric outcome. Little information exists in the literature to understand what level of risk for pregnancy is present for the unsterilized patient postablation with an unsterilized partner. Hill and Maher reported on an uneventful pregnancy following endometrial coagulation and resection (23). Placental pathology revealed a single placental infarct with other nonspecific findings.

Whitelaw and colleagues polled members of the British Society for Gynaecological Endoscopy with ten pregnancies reported (24). Most of these patients chose elective termination, but two patients elected to carry to term. One patient who had undergone Nd-YAG laser ablation had an uncomplicated pregnancy. The second patient, who was 44 years old, had also undergone laser ablation. She was delivered at 39 weeks gestation for breech, intrauterine growth retardation (IUGR), and pregnancy-induced hypertension.

The infant was subsequently diagnosed with single-suture *craniosynostosis* (premature fusion of the cranial vault sutures). In an addendum to Whitelaw's paper, they reported on 16 additional pregnancies in a series of 985 ablations (24). Again, most patients elected for termination. Three patients of the 16 chose to continue their pregnancies. One patient was delivered by cesarean section at 31 weeks for severe IUGR. Placenta increta was noted, for which the patient underwent three subsequent dilations and curettages. In the second patient, placenta accreta necessitated hysterectomy. In the third patient, cesarean section was performed at 29 weeks for severe IUGR and oligohydramnios. The placenta had to be shaved off.

All patients should be counseled that endometrial ablation is not a sterilization procedure. While the exact risk of obstetric complications in patients who conceive after ablative procedures is unknown, patients should be counseled that should they choose not to be sterilized or use a reliable form of contraception, their risk is increased. Frank discussion and documentation is important.

ELECTRICAL AND LASER INJURIES

Injury resulting from the use of electrical energy and its thermal effects is rarely a problem but, when it occurs, can be life-threatening.

Electrical shocks to the patient or to the surgeon from the body of the resectoscope occurred with the early prototypes of the resectoscope, but improvements in design have corrected the problem.

In patients desiring future fertility, thermal injury to the walls of the uterus with resultant scarring is a potential problem that may result from electrical as well as laser energy. Although theoretical, this problem has not been reported and no sequelae appear to occur in the few studies reporting on the efficacy of using laser or electrical (resectoscopic) energy to incise septae. When possible, intrauterine surgery in the patient with intrauterine adhesions should be performed with hysteroscopic scissors to minimize the theoretical risk of excessive scarring inside the uterus due to thermal damage occurring from electrical or laser energy.

Laser or electrical injury to adjacent bowel is almost always due to perforation of the uterus during operative procedures requiring energy. However, a study evaluating efficacy of using a hysteroscopically inserted coagulation electrode into the tubal cornu for the purpose of inducing tubal sterilization was abruptly stopped because of the significant risk of bowel injury, adjacent or adherent to this very thin part of the uterine wall, which resulted in one death and several other cases of bowel damage (25). Caution must be taken not to apply strong electrical or laser energy to these areas for long periods of time. There have been reports of bowel thermal injury occurring during Nd–YAG laser endometrial ablation. Indman and Brown have reported a lack of significant increase in temperature occurring on the serosal surface when a resectoscopic electrode is held against the endometrial surface, using standard power settings, even when held there for up to five seconds (26).

A recent report described full thickness myometrial necrosis with small bowel injury in a patient undergoing endometrial coagulation ablation (27). The patient presented on the second postoperative day and at laparotomy was noted to have an ileal serosal burn and perforation. Interestingly, no area of uterine perforation could be documented on pathologic examination of the hysterectomy specimen.

Sullivan and colleagues reported a case of uterine perforation during resectoscopic resection of a uterine myoma (28). Laparoscopy demonstrated a midline uterine perforation but failed to identify a transmural sigmoid injury secondary to inadequate visualization. Laparotomy and primary repair of the nonprepped sigmoid were performed with no apparent sequelae.

CERVICAL STENOSIS AND HEMATOMETRIA

Another undesirable result is the development of cervical stenosis and or hematometria after endometrial ablation using either laser or electrical energy. This problem can be avoided by being especially careful not to ablate tissue at or below the internal os.

While this has not occurred in our series, it has been noted in several other studies of endometrial ablations, in fewer than 5% of cases, particularly subsequent to the use of the Nd–YAG laser to destroy the endometrium.

Goldrath suggested all patients undergo office suction curettage following Nd–YAG laser ablation (29). He noted 12 cases of postoperative hematometria during these procedures and recommended repeating curettage weekly to decrease the recurrence. It is unclear whether Nd–YAG laser ablation may have a higher incidence of hematometria than coagulation ablation.

Townsend and colleagues described a postablation tubal sterilization syndrome where they noted an association of pelvic pain and vaginal spotting in women who had undergone a previous tubal sterilization and more recent rollerball endometrial ablation (30).

Laparoscopy and hysteroscopy revealed dilated fallopian tubes and scarrified endometrial cavities but patent cornua that were thought to contain endometrial tissue. This may have been a subset of patients with cornual hematometria who are unable to pass endometrial tissue and secretions transtubally secondary to the previous sterilization or transcervically secondary to adhesions.

Ultrasonographic evaluation in patients with symptoms of cyclical pain may help in evaluating the adnexa to rule out hydro- or hematosalpinx and in evaluating the uterine cavity for evidence of fluid collections consistent with hematometria. Goldrath suggested hematometria are unlikely to develop remotely more than 3 months following surgery (29). However, there is a report of a hematometria developing in a patient who was subsequently placed on estrogen replacement therapy (31).

ENDOMETRIAL CANCER

There is the concern that performing endometrial ablations may result in remaining viable endometrial glands that might later undergo malignant change and go undetected until very late. The fear of hiding a subsequent endometrial cancer by performing endometrial ablation is entirely theoretical and has no basis in fact. To begin with, the belief that the entire endometrial cavity is obliterated by scar tissue, much like what may happen in the development of Asherman's syndrome, is not true. We have performed office hysteroscopy for over 30 patients from 4 to 12 months following ablation and have noted a narrow tubular cavity with access to the vagina in every case (see Chapter 13). Goldrath (32) reported the same using serial hysterosalpingography. Furthermore, patients with recurrences of abnormal bleeding even years after ablation present with external bleeding, not unlike patients who have not had ablations.

In addition, in the 15 or more years since the first reports of laser ablation, there has been only one case of endometrial carcinoma reported after an endometrial ablation (33), and that occurred in a patient with a persistent history of adenomatous hyperplasia for eight years prior to the ablation. It may be that endometrial ablation is less appropriate for patients with significant hyperplastic endometrial disease. One reason for the low frequency of later endometrial problems may be that the single layer of cuboidal epithelium we find covering the myometrium in postablation hysterectomy specimens is unresponsive to the endogenous stimuli that induce malignant change.

What is unknown is whether patients will present later in the disease course of endometrial cancer since residual endometrium exists in a significant percent of patients. Most of the 35,000 new cases of endometrial cancer present as Stage I lesions, many with abnormal bleeding. Cervical stenosis could potentially prevent vaginal bleeding and cause delayed diagnosis. This underscores the importance of a patent cervical canal following those procedures. In the one case of an endometrial carcinoma presenting after endometrial ablation, abnormal bleeding through a patent canal allowed rapid diagnosis of the patient's potentially surgically curable early stage lesion.

It is for similar reasons that a combination regimen of estrogen and progestin has been recommended in postmenopausal patients who have previously undergone endometrial ablation by coagulation or resection.

FAILURES AND POOR OUTCOMES

Obviously, the inability of the hysteroscopic surgery to correct the patient's presenting problem may be considered one of the most significant complications.

It is an undesirable outcome when abnormal bleeding is not controlled, the intrauterine synechiae recur or occur de novo following surgery, or if the procedure must be abandoned due to the development of complications, such as perforation of the uterus or fluid overload. Fortunately, these are very uncommon and, in many cases, may be avoided by care and experience.

THE ROLE OF LAPAROSCOPY IN REDUCING THE RISK OF RESECTOSCOPIC SURGERY

Since perforation of the uterus and injury of adjacent organs (bowel, bladder, blood vessels, etc.) are among the most serious complications of operative hysteroscopy, it is often very beneficial to perform concomitant laparoscopy. Although we do not schedule all patients to have laparoscopy at the time of all operative hysteroscopies, we obtain consent for it in all cases, in case it is needed (Table 14-1).

TABLE 14-1

When to Perform Concomitant Laparoscopy

WISE TO *ALWAYS* GET CONSENT

FOR LYSIS OF ADHESIONS
  Always with dense adhesions or total obstruction
  Rarely for isolated or focal adhesions

FOR SEPTOPLASTY
  Always (unless under U.S. monitoring)

FOR ABLATION
  Rarely necessary
  Beginners (?)

FOR MYOMECTOMY
  Rarely for pedunculated tumors
  Maybe for intramural lesions

FOR TUBAL STERILIZATION
  When patient has not solved contraception question
  Perform sterilization *AFTER* ablation or myomectomy is done

WITH PERFORATION
  Always if perforation done with energy source
  If perforation is lateral
  If continued bleeding

Laparoscopy is indicated in the following situations:

- *For lysis of intrauterine adhesions,* laparoscopy should be used when there are lateral dense adhesions or total uterine obstruction, to warn the hysteroscopic surgeon that he or she may be getting dangerously close to the serosal surface. For isolated or focal intrauterine adhesions, laparoscopic monitoring is rarely necessary.
- *For incision of uterine septae,* laparoscopy is helpful in protecting against incising too far and perforating the fundus.
- *For endometrial ablation,* it is rarely necessary, except possibly for beginners. In our experience, after performing laparoscopy during the first 30 ablations, the lack of evidence of getting too deep into the myometrium or producing any thermal change on the serosa left the impression that concomitant laparoscopy was not cost- or risk–effective enough to perform routinely for this procedure.
- *For hysteroscopic myomectomy,* laparoscopy is rarely necessary for pedunculated tumors but, sometimes, may be useful for myomata with a significant intramural component. It is our recommendation that intracavitary sessile myomas be resected hysteroscopically only if more than 50% of the tumor protrudes into the endometrial cavity, and that the resection be carried down only to the level of the concavity of the uterine wall.
- *For tubal sterilization at the time of the hysteroscopic procedure,* the tubal sterilization procedure should be performed at the conclusion of the hysteroscopy so that the intrauterine pressure necessary to achieve adequate uterine distention does not force occluded tubes open.

Laparoscopy is seldom necessary if the perforation of the uterus is in the midline and occurs with blunt instruments, such as uterine sounds or dilators. If the perforation is lateral into the parametrium or occurs with a laser fiber or an electrosurgical electrode, it is almost always necessary to evaluate for damage to adherent or adjacent organs (bowel, bladder, etc.). It is well understood that thermal injury to bowel wall, for example, may result in a slow devitali-

> ## CLINICAL PEARLS
>
> ✖ Complications of operative hysteroscopy are relatively infrequent and often can be prevented if the surgeon is experienced and observes due caution.
>
> ✖ Once you suspect that the patient is in even a little trouble, STOP THE PROCEDURE AND COME BACK ANOTHER TIME!
>
> ✖ Patients get into severe trouble faster than it takes to get into a little trouble!
>
> ✖ Understanding the risks inherent in the use of the instruments and media selected will minimize the chances of complication and enhance the chances of a good surgical result.
>
> ✖ The performance of concomitant laparoscopy in selected cases can help to avoid some of the more severe complications that can occur during operative hysteroscopy.

zation of the tissue and a long delay before breakdown ensues. However, it is almost always essential that the surgeon performs laparoscopy after such perforation to try to detect damage if at all possible.

REFERENCES

1. Survey of American Association of Gynecologic Laparoscopists: Office hysteroscopy, national statistics. 1988 AAGL membership survey. J Reprod Med 1990;35:590–591.
2. Obstetrician connected in sterilization death is placed on probation. Obstet Gynecol News 1974;9:4.
3. Lomano JM, Feste JR, Loffer FD, Goldrath MH. Ablation of the endometrium with the Nd:YAG laser: a multicenter study. Colposc Laser Surg 1986;2:203–207.
4. Goldrath MH, Fuller TA. Intrauterine laser surgery. In: Keye WR,

ed. Laser surgery in gynecology and obstetrics. Boston: GK Hall Medical, 1985;93–110.

5. Serden SP, Brooks PG. Treatment of abnormal uterine bleeding with the gynecologic resectoscope. J Reprod Med 1991;36:697–699.

6. DeCherney AH, Diamond, Lavy G, Polan ML. Endometrial ablation for intractable uterine bleeding: hysteroscopic resection. Obstet Gynecol 1987;70:668–670.

7. Corson SL, Brooks, PG, Serden SP, Batzer FR, Gocial B. The effects of vasopressin administration during hysteroscopic surgery. J Reprod Med 1994;39:419–423.

8. Townsend DE. Vasopressin pack for treatment of bleeding after myoma resection. Am J Obstet Gynecol 1991;165:1405.

9. Brooks PG, Serden SP, Davos I. Hormonal inhibition of the endometrium for resectoscopic endometrial ablation. Am J Obstet Gynecol 1991;164:1601–1608.

10. Brooks PG, Serden SP. Preparation of the endometrium for ablation with a single dose of leuprolide acetate depot. J Reprod Med 1991; 36:477–478.

11. Siegler AM, Valle RF, Lindemann HJ, Mencaglia L. Endometrial ablation. In: Therapeutic hysteroscopy, indications, and techniques. St. Louis: CV Mosby, 1990:149–163.

12. Lindemann HJ, Mohr J, Gallinat A. Der einfluss von CO_2-Gas wahrend der hysteroskopie. Gebrutshilfe Frauendheilkd 1976;36:153–163.

13. Corson SL, Hoffman JJ. Cardiopulmonary effects of direct venous carbon dioxide insufflation. J Reprod Med 1988; 33:440–444.

14. Perry PM, Baughman VL. A complication of hysteroscopy: air embolism. Anesthesiology 1990;73:546–548.

15. Challener RC, Kaufman B. Fatal venous air embolism following sequential unsheathed (bare) and sheathed quartz fiber Nd:YAG laser endometrial ablation. Anesthesiology 1990;73:51–52.

16. FDA bulletin: gas/air embolism associated with intrauterine laser surgery. Washington, D.C., May 1990, 6–7.

17. Renck H. Prevention of dextran-induced anaphylactic reactions. Acta Chir Scand 1983;149:335.

18. Hoekstra PT, Kahnoski R, McCamish MA, Bergen W, Heetdersk DW. Transurethral prostatic resection syndrome—a new perspective: encephalopathy with associated hyperammonemia. J. Urol 1983;130: 704–707.

19. Burkart SS, Barnett CR, Snyder SJ: Transient postoperative blindness as a possible effect of glycine toxicity. Arthroscopy 1990;6:112–114.

20. Salat-Baroux J, Hamou JE, Maillard G. Complications from microhysteroscopy. In: Siegler A, Lindemann JHJ, eds. Hysteroscopy, principles, and practices. Philadelphia: Lippincott, 1984:112–117.

21. McCausland VM, Fields GA, McCausland AM, Townsend DE. Tubo-ovarian abscesses after operative hysteroscopy. J Reprod Med 1993;38:198–200.

22. Cohen MR, Dmowski WP. Modern hysteroscopy. Diagnostic and therapeutic potential. Fertil Steril 1973;24:905–909.

23. Hill DJ, Maher PF. Pregnancy following endometrial ablation. Gynecol Endocrinol 1992;1:47–48.

24. Whitelaw NL, Garry R, Sutton CJG. Pregnancy following endometrial ablation: 2 case reports. Gynecol Endocrinol 1992;1:129–131.

25. Darabi K, Roy K, Richart RM. Collaborative studies on hysteroscopic sterilization procedures: final report. In: Sciarra JJ, Zatuchni GI, Speidel JJ, eds. Risks, benefits, and controversies in fertility control. Hagerstown, Md: Harper and Row, 1978:81–101.

26. Indman PD, Brown WW. Uterine surface temperature changes caused by electrosurgical endometrial coagulation. J Reprod Med 1192;37:667–668.

27. Kivneck S, Kanter MH. Bowel injury from rollerball ablation of the endometrium. Obstet Gynecol 1992;79:883–884.

28. Sullivan B, Kenney P, Siebel M. Hysteroscopic resection of fibroid with thermal injury to sigmoid. Obstet Gynecol 1992;80:546–547.

29. Goldrath MH. Use of danazol in hysteroscopic surgery for menorrhagia. J Reprod Med 1990;35:91–92.

30. Townsend DE, McCausland V, McCausland A, Fields G, Kauffman K. Postablation tubal sterilization syndrome. Obstet Gynecol 1993;82:422–423.

31. Dwyer N, Fox R, Mills M, Hutton J. Haematometra caused by hormone replacement therapy after endometrial resection. Lancet 1991;338:1205–1206.

32. Goldrath MH. Hysteroscopic laser ablation of the endometrium. Obstet Gynecol Forum 1990;4:2–4.

33. Copperman AB, DeCherney AH, Olive DL. A case of endometrial cancer following endometrial ablation for dysfunctional uterine bleeding. Obstet Gynecol 1993;82:640–642.

Index

Ablation, defined, 195
Abortion, repeated, due to intrauterine adhesions, 156
Adenocarcinoma, risk of, and biopsy prior to endometrial ablation, 199
Adenomyoma, anatomy of, 169–170
Adenomyosis
  diagnosis of, 97, 104, 205–206
  hysterectomy for, 99, 189
  and leiomyoma removal, 180, 184
  menometrorrhagia caused by, 95
Adhesions
  intrauterine
    abortion due to, 156
    lysis of, 11, 15, 24, 92, 283
    prediction of, 104
  pelvic, 189
  postoperative, in resection of intrauterine lesions, 182–183
Adrenaline, 227
Alternating current, 49
  radiofrequency, 27–46
Amenorrhea
  comparison of ablation procedures, 119–120
  comparison of endometrial ablation techniques, 58, 241

after electrodesiccation, 210–211
after endometrial ablation, repeat procedure, 261–262
with intrauterine adhesions, 155
ϵ-Aminocaproic acid, for reducing menstrual blood loss, 99
Anaphylactic reaction, Hyskon associated with, 87, 274
Anatomy
  assessment of, by the surgeon, 202–203
  of intrauterine lesions, 169–170
Androgen
  excess, and dysfunctional uterine bleeding, 100
  and symptoms in danocrine use, 113
Anemia
  association with menorrhagia, 95
  and blood transfusion in surgery, 116
  progestins for treating, 112
  and treatment for dysfunctional bleeding, 102
Anesthesia
  in endometrial resection, 226–228
  masking of cerebral edema by, 207
  prior to electrodesiccation, 200

Anesthesia (*cont.*)
  prior to resectoscopic surgery,
    103, 257
Anovulation, and dysfunctional uter-
    ine bleeding, 100, 104
Antibiotics
  for infection complicating elec-
    trodesiccation, 208–209
  prophylactic
    in electrodesiccation, 209
    in excessive uterine bleeding,
      104
    in hysteroscopic surgery, 173,
      223, 276
    after surgery for intrauterine ad-
      hesions, 163–164
Antifibrinolytic agents, systemic, for
    reducing menstrual blood
    loss, 99
Antiprostaglandins, for reducing
    menstrual blood loss, 99
Application time, electrosurgery, and
    tissue damage, 29
Asherman's syndrome, 277, 280
  evaluation of, 93
Atrophy, induced by progestins, 111

Ball electrodes, 15, 197
  for treating bleeding during elec-
    trodesiccation, 208
Ball-end resectoscope, 118
Balloon, for control of uterine bleed-
    ing, 182, 187, 208
Bar/barrel electrode, 15
Bicornuate uterus, 129
Biological changes, due to
    electrosurgery, 53–57
Biophysical considerations,
    electrosurgery, 28–30
Biopsy, endometrial, in evaluating
    menorrhagia, 98

Biopsy, endometrial
  in anovulatory bleeding, 100–101,
    104
  before electrodesiccation, 199
  before endometrial resection, 220–
    221
  malignancy or atypia found by,
    219
  before operative hysteroscopy, 172
  in surgery for uterine septa, 129
Biopsy forceps, in intrauterine adhe-
    sion surgery, 158
Birth control pill. *See* Oral contracep-
    tives
Blanching
  of tissue in electrodesiccation,
    203–204
Bleeding
  abnormal uterine, evaluation of,
    93–94
  dysfunctional uterine, 100–102
  resection of intrauterine lesions
    for, 183
    with endometrial ablation, 190
    hysteroscopic surgery, 171–172
  risk of
    in electrodesiccation, 208
    in endometrial resection, 234
    in resection of intrauterine
      lesions, 182, 187
  and use of carbon dioxide for
    distention, 66
  See also Hemorrhage
Blended current, 51, 177, 226
Blood
  controlling loss of, in surgery,
    109
  miscibility with Hyskon
    distention medium, 72
  mixture with saline, continuous
    flow instrument, 67–68

irrigation fluid, 7
loss to the peritoneum, 76
Gonadotropin-releasing hormone (GnRH)
  agonists to
    evaluation of pretreatment with, 121–122
    pretreatment with, 124, 256
    for reducing menstrual bleeding, 99, 114, 119
    for shrinking leiomyomas, 264
    preparation for electrodesiccation, 199–200
  analogs
    for postoperative endometrial suppression, 240
    pretreatment with, 221, 233
    proposed postoperative treatment with, 124
  side effects of, 112
Goserelin acetate. *See* Gonadotropin-releasing hormone (GnRH), agonists to
Growths. *See* Intrauterine lesions; Leiomyomata; Myoma; Polyps

Hazards. *See* Safety considerations
Heat
  and current density, 51–52
  and electrosurgical damage, 33–34
Hematometra, 279–280
  after endometrial ablation, 244
Hematoxylin and eosin (H&E) stain, 31, 59
  demonstration of electrocautery damage, 36
Hemoglobin
  effect on levels, by GnRHa, 115
  increasing levels of, prior to surgery, 109

Hemolysis, caused by water distention medium, 68
Hemorrhage
  in operative hysteroscopy, 271–273
  peripheral to electrosurgical burns, 39–41, 46
  risk of
    in endometrial resection, 236, 240
    in resection of intrauterine lesions, 182
  See also Bleeding
Hemostasis, and choice of current, 226
Histology
  in electrodesiccation, 199
  of electrosurgical damage, 33–45
  in endometrial resection, 234
  of hysterectomy specimens, 58
Hormonal manipulation, conditioning the endometrium prior to electrodesiccation, 199–200
Hormonal treatment, postoperative, 163–164, 209
Hot spots, in electrocautery, 35
21-Hydroxylase deficiency, and androgen excess, 100
Hyperammonemia, from glycine metabolism, 70
Hyperplasia
  atypical, 219
    and risk of carcinoma after endometrial resection, 245–246
  endometrial, and chronic anovulation, 100–101
  and risk of carcinoma after endometrial resection, 281
Hypertension, in postTUR syndrome, 79
Hypertonicity, of Hyskon, 87

Ovarian failure, premature
dysfunctional uterine bleeding as a
sign of, 100
following hysterectomy, 238
Oviducts, rupturing, from excessive
gas pressures, 270
Oxycodene, 183
Oxygen, use with respiratory depressant anesthetics, 227

Pain
after electrodesiccation, 209–210
after endometrial ablation, 244,
280
hysterectomy for, 189
related to endometriosis, 196–197,
212
after resection of intrauterine
lesions, 183
Panoramic field, telescopic, 16–17
Paramesonephric ducts, origin of
uterus in, 128
Pathologists, examination of
electrosurgical damage by,
30–31
Pedunculated growth, defined, 169–
170
Pedunculization, of fibroids, 178
Pelvic inflammatory disease (PID),
173, 276
Peritoneal fluid, glycine leaked to, in
transcervical endometrial
resection, 76
Peritonitis, following electrodesiccation, 210
Perivascular damage, from
electrocautery, 46
Picrosirius red stain, for assessing
electrosurgical damage, 32
Pitressin, administration in surgery,
182, 201, 272–273

Pituitary rongeur, 22
Platelets
abnormalities of, in menorrhagia,
97
effect on, of Hyskon, 87
Point-tip electrode, 15
for uterine adhesion surgery, 161
Polycystic ovary syndrome, dysfunctional uterine bleeding with,
100
Polypectomy, 168–191
carbon dioxide use in, 67
resectoscopic technique, 177–178
Polyps
endometrial, 169–170
menometrorrhagia caused by, 95
large, resectoscopes suitable for removal of, 11, 24
loop electrode device for removal
of, 15
preoperative identification of, 191,
220–221
removal of, 98–99
small, resectoscopes suitable for removal of, 11, 24
Polyp snares, 172–173
Postablation tubal sterilization syndrome, 279–280
Postoperative treatment, 122–125
with DMPA, 124
in electrodesiccation, 209–210
for endometrial ablation, repeat
procedure, 260
in endometrial resection, 240
after leiomyoma resection, 265–
266
resection of intrauterine lesions,
183
PostTUR syndrome, 79
Power
delivery to tissue, 176

Provera. *See* Depomedroxyprogesterone acetate
Pseudodecidual changes
induced by progestins, 111
Pulmonary embolus, possibility of,
in distention with carbon
dioxide, 66–67
Pyelogram, intravenous, screening,
131

Radiofrequency (RF) currents
effects on tissue, 27–46
path of, 34–35
Rate of electrodesiccation, and adequacy of ablation, 205
Reepithelialization, after intrauterine
adhesion surgery, 163–164
Refractive index
of carbon dioxide, 66
ideal, for distention medium, 63
of normal saline solutions, 67
Renal anomalies, associated with uterine septa, 131
Renal damage, from inappropriate
distention media, 68
Renal excretion, of Hyskon, 84–85
Reproductive outcome
of hysteroscopic treatment of uterine adhesions, 164–165
of hysteroscopic treatment of uterine septa, 146–147
Reproductive outcomes. *See also*
Pregnancy
Reproductive problems, 155. *See also*
Infertility
Resecting loop
shaving the endometrium with,
48
Resection
defined, 195

versus electrodesiccation, estimating end-point in, 199–200
partial, defined, 233
Resectoscopes
continuous flow, 172–173, 215
for debris removal, 177
for electrodesiccation, 201
list, 12
with cutting loop, for treatment
of uterine septa, 147
for division
of intrauterine adhesions, 161–
162
of intrauterine adhesions, results, 164
of uterine septa, 137–142
effective use of, 234–235
gynecologic, instrumentation, 9–
16, 23, 223–224
historic perspective, 1–8
for myomectomy, 262, 265
for removal of intrauterine lesions, 172–173
repeat procedures using, 254–266
techniques for using,
myomectomy and
polypectomy, 173–180
urological single-flow, 215
Resistance, 48
and coagulation waveforms, 55
and tissue desiccation, 56
Reticuloendothelial system, loss of
Hyskon particles through,
84–85
Retractors, vaginal wall, 21
Ringer's solution, lactated, for
distention, 67–68, 87, 136,
158–159, 162–163, 225, 257
Risks, of leiomyoma resection, 263–
265. *See also* Safety considerations